Lord, why am I ill?

Lord, why am I ill?

Why Christians fall ill –
and how all illness can be healed

And the LORD said unto him, Who hath made man's
mouth? or who maketh the dumb, or deaf, or the seeing, or
the blind? have not I the LORD? (Exodus 4:11)

Tom Harrison

Rickfords Hill Publishing Ltd.

Published by
RICKFORDS HILL PUBLISHING LTD.
P.O. Box 576, Aylesbury, Buckinghamshire HP22 6XX, UK.

First published 2008

ISBN 978-1-905044-04-7

Printed and bound in China by 1010 Printing International Ltd.

Contents

SECTION I

SECTION II – Guidance Notes

Acknowledgements

The author would like to express his sincere thanks to Dr Jeremy Boucher for comments and suggestions on medical factual accuracy. Any mistakes are the author's own.

SECTION I

He healeth me

He healeth me, O blessèd truth,
His mighty word renews my youth,
By His own power from sickness free,
My precious Saviour healeth me.

He healeth me, He healeth me,
By His own word He healeth me;
His faithful witness I would be,
For by His word He healeth me.

Sometimes through testing times I go,
Dark seems the way, and full of woe;
But in the furnace though I be,
My great Physician healeth me.

Lord, I would spread this truth abroad,
The mighty power of Thy word;
It's just the same, the blind now see,
And demons at Thy presence flee.

For sin and sickness doth depart,
When Thou dost reign within the heart;
And I from all the curse am free,
Since Christ, my Saviour, healeth me.

Anonymous, from Redemption Hymnal

1

A testimony

In the spring of 2003 I was busy serving the Lord. I was in church leadership and at the same time was running a Christian publishing company. I was seeking to be all out for God. Then I fell ill.

What started as a virus turned into a particularly bad case of *systemic candidiasis*. This is an unpleasant disease in which a fungus, *candida albicans*, lives in your digestive system, feeds on the food you eat and then releases toxins into your blood stream, which then poison the rest of your body. The symptoms are diarrhoea, aching muscles, chronic fatigue, mental incoherence and others.

I was unable to do much work as a result of this illness and I had to lie on my bed most of the day from exhaustion. Diarrhoea was a part of daily life. If I ate a normal meal, within half an hour my body would be racked with aches, and my mind as incoherent as if I were drunk.

I found, however, that by following a strict diet I could get some relief. This diet consisted of only potatoes, oil, meat and fish. I kept to this as much as I could but every few days I had to eat some other things, such as fruit, in order to stop myself feeling ill from malnutrition. This however made me feel ill again from the candidiasis.

This lasted for two and a half years.

When I first became ill, I was wondering if there was any

reason for it. I meditated on it and the passage of scripture that
came to mind was this:

> And as Jesus passed by, he saw a man which was blind from
> his birth. And his disciples asked him, saying, Master, who did
> sin, this man, or his parents, that he was born blind? Jesus
> answered, Neither hath this man sinned, nor his parents.
> (John 9:1-3)

I thought that this was the Lord's answer to my question, so from
that point on I didn't look for a reason for my illness. I just trusted
God to use my life as He chose, even if this meant I had to endure
physical illness. I thought that the Lord might want me to suffer
just for the general refinement of my character.

After two and a half years I was desperate to be healed. I
had been to three GPs, a consultant haematologist, a consultant
dermatologist, a consultant gastroenterologist, had had four
courses of drugs, numerous blood tests, had tried many different
herbal remedies and supplements, but felt as bad as I had ever
done.

Through all this I was continuing to seek to maintain a close
walk with God. One day, as I was communing with the Lord, I
was asking Him what I could do to walk more closely with Him,
and how I could please Him. I felt Him say, 'It saddens me that
you go to earthly doctors and not to me.'

A few days later I heard my brother preach a gospel message
on the woman with the issue of blood.

> And a certain woman, which had an issue of blood twelve
> years, and had suffered many things of many physicians,
> and had spent all that she had, and was nothing bettered, but
> rather grew worse, when she had heard of Jesus, came in the
> press behind, and touched his garment. For she said, If I may
> touch but his clothes, I shall be whole. And straightway the
> fountain of her blood was dried up; and she felt in her body that
> she was healed of that plague. (Mark 5:25-29)

I was struck by the fact that the doctors, as in my case, had been
unable to help her. I felt challenged again that I should be getting

my healing from the Lord. However, I had been out for prayer in two churches. Elders had laid hands on me and prayed. I was no better. I didn't know what to do.

Over a period of some weeks, I started drawing very near to the Lord. I cut out every kind of distraction from my life. Then I was asked to give a message at a church's Prayer and Bible Week. I sought the Lord for a message, and He gave me something I had never heard or understood before, a message about discerning the body of Christ.

The heart of the message was that God has provided His church (the body of Christ) for our spiritual food, and that by spending time with other believers we are fed spiritually. Consequently, we should not despise any part of it and should realise how precious it is, love it, enjoy it, cherish it, and treat it with the respect it deserves. This includes every believer, whatever his failings, and every church of every denomination (this obviously refers only to born again people – the true church).

This completely changed my outlook. I had known that my personal fellowship with God was my spiritual food, but I had not seen my need for fellowship with people. I had been choosy about whom I would associate with, dismissing individuals and churches; I had only been interested in my own personal encounter with God rather than enjoying fellowship with other believers. The Lord made it clear to me that fellowship with other people was part of my spiritual diet. *(For more on this subject see* Digestive System*, page 148).*

In the period preceding this I had kept rigidly to the exclusion diet, eating only meat, fish, oil and potatoes. I ate absolutely nothing else for several weeks. At the end of this period I felt so continually hungry that it made me feel 'spiritually hungry' at the same time. I just had a desire for everything and especially for the fellowship of others.

The Prayer and Bible Week was an intense time spiritually. I came back home exhausted, but immediately felt strongly impressed to fast for a few days. On the third day of my fast, I prayed that I would have the faith for my healing.

The next day I was seeking the Lord for something else, and

suddenly I felt strongly that God really wanted to heal me. I always knew He could, but suddenly I realised that my heavenly Father wanted to give me good things and not to have me suffer unnecessarily. I asked Him to heal me. In response, He powerfully revealed to me that my healing was to be found in the wounds of the Lord Jesus and nowhere else.

> With his stripes we are healed. (Isaiah 53:5)

After a few seconds of seeing this truth, I suddenly had the impression 'I have received my healing', and had the sensation not of healing but of cleansing sweeping through my body. I felt cleansed, washed, and came into a sense of rest. As I relaxed I felt full of joy and was certain that I had been healed. Indeed it proved to be so. The candida had entirely gone.

I realized through all this that I had been wrong at the outset, that my illness *had* been the result of sin: it had been God's way of revealing it to me and correcting me. If I had known this at the beginning, my healing might have come far more quickly and easily.

Since being healed myself, the Lord has opened up for me the whole subject in a remarkable way, showing the link between sin and sickness, so that I can now say with certainty that all sickness reveals to us a problem in our spiritual condition. My purpose in writing this book is to help reveal to others what it took me so long to understand, that their healing might come quickly and easily, and that God might be glorified.

2

Lord, why am I ill?

All things in the life of a believer happen for a purpose.

> And we know that all things work together for good to them
> that love God, to them who are the called according to his
> purpose. (Romans 8:28)

There is no single event that happens to us without the Lord's
allowing it. We must assume then that all illness is given to us
for a specific purpose. Why then does God allow His children to
become ill?

As we look through the Bible we find that there is an undeniable
link between sickness and sin. It is God's loudhailer, trying to
break through to our consciousness that something is wrong. It
started in the Garden of Eden when man first fell. And just as
sickness came onto the whole human race to alert it to the fact
that it had fallen into sin, so sickness in the body of an individual
believer is God's way of alerting him to some area of failing in
his life.

As we look into the subject more closely, we discover that God
gives specific sicknesses to highlight specific sins.

It may cause us some alarm to think that our sickness is caused
by sin, but really it should cause us to rejoice because once the

sin is dealt with, healing can come easily. It should also please us to know that God has provided us with such an obvious way of knowing that something is wrong in our lives. After all, as believers, our chief aim should be to live in a way that pleases the Lord.

Since it is not widely taught, this truth may also make us worried that this is some new unbiblical doctrine that is being propagated. It is, however, absolutely biblical, as we trust will be shown. Indeed, in the Lord's time on earth, it was generally believed, but has now largely been forgotten.

Understanding and applying this teaching will not only bring healing to the individual but will also help us to deal with sins in our lives, leading us on a path of spiritual growth. We need, therefore, to study the scriptures to see what they really say about sickness and healing.

Before continuing

One final thing that is necessary before continuing is to gain a correct understanding of sin. Some people are very frightened of the word 'sin' and think that it only means gross offences like murder and adultery. In reality, it is any kind of failing, and it is part of our fallen nature.

Romans 3:23 states that 'all have sinned, and come short of the glory of God.' We therefore take sin to be anything that

- falls short of God's perfection and therefore
- displeases God and therefore
- needs to be corrected.

Although this includes things such as adultery and fornication, it also includes things that are not commonly thought to be sins but which the Lord doesn't want to see in us. Examples of these are

- Worry (not trusting the Lord)
- Carrying our burdens (not casting them on the Lord)
- Bringing things up from the past
- Not listening to the Lord – or other people

- Not being diligent in Christian service
- Being small-minded

As human beings, we are born sinners and continue to be sinners until the day we die. Even as Christians, we are redeemed, justified and ready for heaven, but while on this earth we still retain the old sinful nature. It is simply the condition we are all in. The Apostle Paul says,

> I am carnal, sold under sin. For that which I do I allow not: for what I would, that do I not; but what I hate, that do I. (Romans 7:14-15)

As we go through our Christian lives, God gradually puts to death the old nature so that the life of Christ, with all His righteousness, can increasingly be displayed in us. Yet in ourselves, there is never anything good. The only righteousness we ever have is Christ's imputed righteousness. Again, Paul says,

> For I know that in me (that is, in my flesh,) dwelleth no good thing. (Romans 7:18)

If, then, we are all sinners, 'sold under sin' and in ourselves utterly devoid of good, it should not surprise us to know that there is sin (things that need correcting), not only in our own lives, but also in the lives of those we love, and in the lives of great men of God.

We should not as Christians be afraid to admit our sins. All sin brings us into bondage so we should want to be free from every sign of it. By admitting it and confessing it we can get right with God, and be brought into glorious liberty.

> If we say that we have no sin, we deceive ourselves, and the truth is not in us. If we confess our sins, he is faithful and just to forgive us our sins, and to cleanse us from all unrighteousness. (I John 1:8, 9)

3

Sin and sickness – What the Bible says

Throughout the Bible, beginning in Genesis and continuing through to the end of the New Testament, God teaches that sickness is given by Him in response to sin. The connection between sin and sickness is both taught and demonstrated again and again, and so we need to begin by tracing how the Lord reveals this truth and makes it plain.

A. The Fall

The first reference we have in the Bible to sickness comes as the Lord God explains the consequences of Adam and Eve's sin. He says to Satan:

> And I will put enmity between thee and the woman, and between thy seed and her seed; it shall bruise thy head, and thou shalt bruise his heel. (Genesis 3:15)

God says that as a result of the fall, mankind will receive physical suffering from Satan ('thou shalt bruise his heel'). He also says that the offspring of the woman will overcome Satan (wounding his head).

The fulness of this prophecy takes place at the cross where

Satan's head is bruised (he is defeated and mortally wounded though not yet finally destroyed) and the Lord Jesus Christ (the seed of the woman) receives suffering, including physical pain and the literal wounding/bruising of His feet. Yet the verse clearly indicates that Satan will inflict physical suffering on all humans as well as upon Christ: the enmity is both between the seed of the woman and the seed of the devil, and between the devil and the woman herself.[1] The principle has been established: sin has brought physical pain onto humans.

The Lord goes on to say to the woman:

> I will greatly multiply thy **sorrow** and thy conception; in **sorrow** thou shalt bring forth children; and thy desire shall be to thy husband, and he shall rule over thee. (Genesis 3.16).

The word translated 'sorrow' can equally mean 'pain'; indeed, the American Standard Version translates it as 'pain' in both cases, and other reputable versions do so in at least one case.

The same Hebrew word is used in reference to Adam:

> Cursed is the ground for thy sake; in **sorrow** shalt thou eat of it all the days of thy life; thorns also and thistles shall it bring forth to thee; (Genesis 3:17, 18)

Again we see that sin has brought physical pain to mankind. Few Christians would disagree with this, but what evidence is there from Scripture that sickness in the individual is caused by that person's sin?

B. God states specifically that sickness is a consequence of sin.

In Deuteronomy 28, after reiterating the law to the Israelites, Moses explains to them the consequences of not obeying the Lord. One of these effects is physical sickness.

---

[1] The fact that all humans are included in this statement as well as Christ is evident from Romans 16:20.

But it shall come to pass, if thou wilt not hearken unto the voice of the LORD thy God, to observe to do all his commandments and his statutes which I command thee this day; that all these curses shall come upon thee, and overtake thee:

The LORD shall make the pestilence cleave unto thee, until he have consumed thee from off the land, whither thou goest to possess it. The LORD shall smite thee with a consumption, and with a fever, and with an inflammation, and with an extreme burning, and with the sword, and with blasting, and with mildew; and they shall pursue thee until thou perish.

The LORD will smite thee with the botch of Egypt, and with the emerods, and with the scab, and with the itch, whereof thou canst not be healed. The LORD shall smite thee with madness, and blindness, and astonishment of heart:

The LORD shall smite thee in the knees, and in the legs, with a sore botch that cannot be healed, from the sole of thy foot unto the top of thy head.

Then the LORD will make thy plagues wonderful, and the plagues of thy seed, even great plagues, and of long continuance, and sore sicknesses, and of long continuance. Moreover he will bring upon thee all the diseases of Egypt, which thou wast afraid of; and they shall cleave unto thee. Also every sickness, and every plague, which is not written in the book of this law, them will the LORD bring upon thee, until thou be destroyed. (Deuteronomy 28:15, 21-22, 27-28, 35, 59-61)

It is made quite clear that a consequence of failing to keep all the commandments of the Lord is physical sickness.

C. Sickness given in response to sin in the Old Testament

Just as God has warned that sickness is a consequence of sin, on a number of occasions we see this demonstrated. In various passages in the Old Testament, it is specifically stated that sickness has come upon an individual as a result of sin. It may be useful to list a good number of these.

♦ When King Uzziah became strong and was lifted up with pride, he went into the temple to burn incense, a role that only the consecrated priesthood could perform. In spite of the priests withstanding him, Uzziah persisted.

> Then Uzziah was wroth, and had a censer in his hand to burn incense: and while he was wroth with the priests, the leprosy even rose up in his forehead before the priests in the house of the LORD, from beside the incense altar. And Azariah the chief priest, and all the priests, looked upon him, and, behold, he was leprous in his forehead, and they thrust him out from thence; yea, himself hasted also to go out, because the LORD had smitten him. (II Chronicles 26:18-20).

The leprosy is given as a result of his sin. (A similar story is also found regarding Miriam and Aaron in Numbers 12.)

♦ We see a similar thing with Jeroboam, when he tries to seize a man of God: his hand is made to wither as a result of his infamous act.

> And it came to pass, when king Jeroboam heard the saying of the man of God, which had cried against the altar in Bethel, that he put forth his hand from the altar, saying, Lay hold on him. And his hand, which he put forth against him, dried up, so that he could not pull it in again to him. (I Kings 13:4).

♦ In response to King Jehoram's wicked reign in which he slew his brothers and led the people astray, the Lord through the prophet Elijah says:

> Because thou hast not walked in the ways of Jehoshaphat thy father, nor in the ways of Asa king of Judah, But hast walked in the way of the kings of Israel, and hast made Judah and the inhabitants of Jerusalem to go a whoring, like to the whoredoms of the house of Ahab, and also hast slain thy brethren of thy father's house, which were better than thyself: Behold, with a great plague will the LORD smite thy people, and thy children, and thy wives, and all thy goods: And thou shalt have great

sickness by disease of thy bowels, until thy bowels fall out by reason of the sickness day by day. (II Chronicles 21)

♦ When Jacob would not submit to the Lord, the Lord brought him to his knees by smiting his hip:

And when he saw that he prevailed not against him, he touched the hollow of his thigh; and the hollow of Jacob's thigh was out of joint, as he wrestled with him. (Genesis 32:25).

♦ When King Nebuchadnezzar is filled with pride, boasting, 'Is not this great Babylon, that I have built for the house of the kingdom by the might of my power, and for the honour of my majesty?', the Lord responds:

O king Nebuchadnezzar, to thee it is spoken; The kingdom is departed from thee. And they shall drive thee from men, and thy dwelling shall be with the beasts of the field: they shall make thee to eat grass as oxen, and seven times shall pass over thee, until thou know that the most High ruleth in the kingdom of men, and giveth it to whomsoever he will. The same hour was the thing fulfilled upon Nebuchadnezzar: and he was driven from men, and did eat grass as oxen, and his body was wet with the dew of heaven, till his hairs were grown like eagles' feathers, and his nails like birds' claws. (Daniel 4:31-33)

♦ In I Samuel 5 it speaks of the Lord smiting the Philistines in response to their taking away the Ark of the Covenant and putting it into the house of the god Dagon:

When the Philistines took the ark of God, they brought it into the house of Dagon, and set it by Dagon. But the hand of the LORD was heavy upon them of Ashdod, and he destroyed them, and smote them with emerods, even Ashdod and the coasts thereof. (I Samuel 5:6)

Again, the Lord's smiting of the Philistines with haemorrhoids is entirely attributed to their sin in removing the Ark.

D. Sickness given in response to sin in the New Testament

Just as in the Old Testament, so in the New, we find sickness given as a result of specific sins.

♦ Zacharias, the father of John the Baptist, when told that he in his old age would have a son, doubted and questioned the angel Gabriel. In response, Gabriel says:

> Behold, thou shalt be dumb, and not able to speak, until the day that these things shall be performed, because thou believest not my words, which shall be fulfilled in their season. (Luke 1:20).

Zacharias was struck dumb entirely because of his attitude towards the word of God.

♦ Even after the Lord's death, resurrection and ascension, we find that the doctrine still holds true. Paul says to the Corinthians

> For he that eateth and drinketh unworthily, eateth and drinketh damnation to himself, not discerning the Lord's body. For this cause many are weak and sickly among you, and many sleep. (I Corinthians 11:29-30)

Clearly a number of believers in the Corinthian church were falling ill and some were dying because they were not 'discerning the Lord's body' *(for a fuller explanation of this passage and what it means to discern the Lord's body, please see page 150ff).*

Again, in Acts 8 when Elymas the sorcerer tries to thwart the work of God, he is made blind:

> The hand of the Lord is upon thee, and thou shalt be blind, not seeing the sun for a season. And immediately there fell on him a mist and a darkness; and he went about seeking some to lead him by the hand. (Acts 13:11)[2]

---

[2] The reason he is made blind is very interesting. He was trying to lead Sergius Paulus away from God. Jesus said, 'Can the blind lead the blind? shall they not both fall into the ditch?' (Luke 6:39) Thus the blindness was being given to show what Elymas was doing spiritually.

So we find that the Lord not only clearly warns that sickness is a consequence of sin, but He gives practical demonstrations of the doctrine in both the Old Testament and New.

E. Sin linked with sickness within the context of healing

Under both the Old Covenant and the New, God has provided a means by which His people can be healed. In the Old Testament, after God's people have been delivered from Egypt and seen a whole nation smitten by disease, God makes it plain to them that by obeying Him and keeping themselves from sin, they can be free from disease. He says,

> If thou wilt diligently hearken to the voice of the LORD thy God, and wilt do that which is right in his sight, and wilt give ear to his commandments, and keep all his statutes, I will put none of these diseases upon thee, which I have brought upon the Egyptians: for I am the LORD that healeth thee. (Exodus 15:26)

Although sickness has come upon man because of sin, the Lord says that by keeping His commandments, they can be free from sin and therefore from the consequences of sin, including disease. This is God's provision of healing under the Old Covenant. Yet, as we know, the Old Covenant was imperfect, because people were unable to keep the law.

When we come to the New Testament, we find that the connection between sin and sickness is still there. What has changed is that the ability to live lives that are free from sin comes by grace. When we become Christians, we come to God in repentance and faith, and He forgives us and gives us the power to live lives that are free from sin. As long as we walk by faith, we abide in the righteousness of Christ, and we are able to live without sinning. By this New Covenant God has enabled His people to be free from sin and therefore free from disease. (It is only as we cease to walk by faith and start to live in the flesh (returning to the old sinful nature) that we start to sin and become ill).

Therefore we see on certain occasions when the Lord Jesus healed people that he highlighted the connection between healing of sickness and forgiveness of sins.

♦ In Matthew 9 we read about a paralytic being brought to Jesus.

> And, behold, they brought to him a man sick of the palsy, lying on a bed: and Jesus seeing their faith said unto the sick of the palsy; Son, be of good cheer; thy sins be forgiven thee. And, behold, certain of the scribes said within themselves, This man blasphemeth. And Jesus knowing their thoughts said, Wherefore think ye evil in your hearts? For whether is easier, to say, Thy sins be forgiven thee; or to say, Arise, and walk? But that ye may know that the Son of man hath power on earth to forgive sins, (then saith he to the sick of the palsy,) Arise, take up thy bed, and go unto thine house. And he arose, and departed to his house. (Matthew 9:2-7)

The Lord's response is very revealing. When the man is brought to be healed, the Lord says 'thy sins be forgiven thee.' But in order to show the people that He has 'power on earth to forgive sins', he says, 'Arise, take up thy bed, and go unto thine house.' In other words, to heal, He forgives, and in order to show that the man is forgiven, He heals. Moreover, he states that telling the man he is forgiven and telling him he is healed amounts to the same thing.

> For whether is easier, to say, Thy sins be forgiven thee; or to say, Arise, and walk?

♦ In John 5, we read of the healing of a wasted man at the pool of Bethesda.

> And a certain man was there, which had an infirmity thirty and eight years. When Jesus saw him lie, and knew that he had been now a long time in that case, he saith unto him, Wilt thou be made whole? The impotent man answered him, Sir, I have no man, when the water is troubled, to put me into the pool: but while I am coming, another steppeth down before

me. Jesus saith unto him, Rise, take up thy bed, and walk. And immediately the man was made whole, and took up his bed, and walked. (John 5:5-9)

There is no mention of sin at the time of the healing. However, the Lord finds him later and speaks to him about the healing:

Afterward Jesus findeth him in the temple, and said unto him, Behold, thou art made whole: sin no more, lest a worse thing come unto thee. (John 5:14).

John Wesley comments:

It seems his former illness was the effect or punishment of sin.[3]

Of course, the Lord Jesus healed many hundreds of other people and the connection between sin and sickness is not always mentioned in Scripture. But just because it isn't stated, it does not mean that forgiveness was not part of the healing.[4]

♦ Another New Testament reference to the connection between sin and sickness in healing is found in James 5.

Is any sick among you? let him call for the elders of the church; and let them pray over him, anointing him with oil in the name of the Lord: and the prayer of faith shall save the sick, and the Lord shall raise him up; and if he have committed sins, they shall be forgiven him. Confess your faults one to another, and pray one for another, that ye may be healed. The effectual fervent prayer of a righteous man availeth much. (James 5:15-16)

This time the healing is within the context of the local church and, again, healing and forgiveness of sins go together. It states first of all that a sick man may be healed when elders pray over him

---

[3] *Wesley's Notes on the Bible*
[4] To argue that because it is not mentioned, it didn't happen, is known as an 'argument from silence' – an unsound method of biblical interpretation.

and his sins are confessed and forgiven. It is also made clear that confessing of faults and mutual prayer amongst believers in general brings healing. Clearly, it is the dealing with sins that opens the way for healing.

Some would suggest that the word 'if' raises a doubt as to whether the person has actually committed sin. The Greek does not bear this out. The sentence can be accurately translated 'and though he has committed sins, they shall be forgiven him.'[5] I believe, therefore, that James is not doubting whether the man has sinned, but is rather laying stress on the wonderful grace of God that is available: 'even though sickness comes from sin, yet God's goodness – in forgiving and healing – is still available.' *(For more on the role of Elders in healing see Chapter 9, page 71).*

So we see that one of the blessings of the New Covenant is that, because sin can be dealt with, the associated sickness can also be removed.

F. The link between sin and sickness at the Cross

We may also ask ourselves the question, 'Why was it that the Lord Jesus had to suffer physical pain in paying the price for our sins?' Sin is a spiritual problem, so was it not enough that He should pay spiritually?

That the Lord Jesus paid for our sins spiritually is clear. He suffered the abandonment of God the Father, crying, 'My God, my God, why hast thou forsaken me?' (Mark 15:34). Psalm 22 and Isaiah 53 describe prophetically something of the spiritual suffering of the Lord.

My God, my God, why hast thou forsaken me? why art thou so far from helping me, and from the words of my roaring? O my

---

[5] In John 8:14, the Lord Jesus uses the same Greek construction, but there it is translated 'though': 'Though I bear record of myself, yet my record is true'. A conditional sentence does not mean there is necessarily any doubt as to the fulfilment of the condition. Cf. I Cor 9:16; II Cor. 10:8; II Cor. 12:6. Indeed, James 5:15 could equally be translated 'Whatever sins he has committed shall be forgiven him'. Cf. Matt. 16:19; Matt 18:18; Gal. 6:7; Eph. 6:8

> God, I cry in the daytime, but thou hearest not; and in the night
> season, and am not silent.
> Be not far from me; for trouble is near; for there is none to help.
> Many bulls have compassed me: strong bulls of Bashan have
> beset me round.
> But be not thou far from me, O LORD: O my strength, haste
> thee to help me. Deliver my soul from the sword; my darling
> from the power of the dog. Save me from the lion's mouth: for
> thou hast heard me from the horns of the unicorns. (Psalm
> 22:1, 2, 11-13, 19-21)

And yet so often when the spiritual sufferings of the Lord Jesus are
described they are coupled together with the physical sufferings.

> He is despised and rejected of men; a man of sorrows, and
> acquainted with grief: and we hid as it were our faces from
> him; he was despised, and we esteemed him not. Surely
> he hath borne our griefs [literally, *diseases*], and carried our
> sorrows [or *pains*]: yet we did esteem him stricken, smitten of
> God, and afflicted. (Isaiah 53:3, 4)

The spiritual and physical terms seem to be used interchangeably.
Why is that?

It is surely because the physical body reflects what is happening
spiritually. So when the Lord Jesus bore 'our sins in his own body
on the tree' (I Peter 2:24), His body was smitten as He bore the
physical pain associated with those sins. Thus the passage from
Isaiah continues,

> He was wounded for our transgressions, he was bruised for
> our iniquities. (Isaiah 53:5)

If the Lord Jesus had never suffered physically, we would have
found it very difficult to grasp that He had suffered spiritually.
The body is like a window into the spiritual life, showing what is
going on there. Sin in the soul brings suffering in the body.

So in the suffering of the Lord Jesus at the cross we see there
is again a link between sin and physical suffering.

G. Scriptures that seem to deny the connection

We have seen again and again in Scripture that sickness is clearly attributed to sin. But what about those passages that would appear to teach the opposite?

1. Paul's thorn in the flesh

Some would argue that Paul had an illness that God would not remove. Let's look at what the Apostle says.

> For though I would desire to glory, I shall not be a fool; for I will say the truth: but now I forbear, lest any man should think of me above that which he seeth me to be, or that he heareth of me. And lest I should be exalted above measure through the abundance of the revelations, there was given to me a thorn in the flesh, the messenger of Satan to buffet me, lest I should be exalted above measure.
>
> For this thing I besought the Lord thrice, that it might depart from me. And he said unto me, My grace is sufficient for thee: for my strength is made perfect in weakness.
>
> Most gladly therefore will I rather glory in my infirmities, that the power of Christ may rest upon me. Therefore I take pleasure in infirmities, in reproaches, in necessities, in persecutions, in distresses for Christ's sake: for when I am weak, then am I strong. (II Corinthians 12:6-10)

The Apostle Paul has been given such tremendous revelations that God says he needs something to keep him humble. Paul describes this as a thorn in the flesh. For generations people have discussed what the 'thorn in the flesh' actually is. Some have thought it to be a physical illness. Others have seen it to be some kind of temptation. However, Paul specifically says what the thorn is: 'the messenger of Satan'. It is a satanic angel or demon.[6]

---

[6] A mere 26 verses earlier, he has referred to Satan appearing as 'an angel of light'. The Greek for *angel* and *messenger* are the same. The word is never used in the New Testament in any other way than to describe a human or angelic messenger (Satanic or Divine). The idea that Paul should suddenly use it as a metaphor for something else here is unsustainable. Cf. Matt. 25:41; Rev. 12:7, 9.

Paul is saying that, because of the revelations he has received, God has allowed a demon to stick by him – to harass him, to buffet or pummel him and to cause him continual difficulties of every kind. The whole purpose of this is to keep Paul weak and trusting in the Lord.

Paul goes on to describe the things that he receives from the demon: infirmities, reproaches, necessities, persecutions, distresses. As he continues to minister, he suffers a barrage of assaults that keep him weak and humble.

In the previous chapter Paul has been listing some of the things that he has suffered for the name of Christ:

> Of the Jews five times received I forty stripes save one. Thrice was I beaten with rods, once was I stoned, thrice I suffered shipwreck, a night and a day I have been in the deep; In journeyings often, in perils of waters, in perils of robbers, in perils by mine own countrymen, in perils by the heathen, in perils in the city, in perils in the wilderness, in perils in the sea, in perils among false brethren... (II Corinthians 11:24-26).

Now as he comes into chapter 12 he explains why he has to endure such suffering: it is to keep him humble.

It is this continual pummelling by a demon, then, that Paul has to be content to accept. He asks the Lord three times to take it away, but the Lord says that it has to stay.

It is important to realise, therefore, that the thorn in the flesh is not a physical illness (though it does cause him physical pain in other ways, such as through persecution), but rather an actual evil spirit. To confirm this, we need to understand more fully what Paul means by the term 'thorn in the flesh'.

Paul is most likely quoting from Numbers 33, where the phrase 'thorn in your sides' is a metaphor for the continual troubling caused by Israel's enemies.

> But if ye will not drive out the inhabitants of the land from before you; then it shall come to pass, that those which ye let remain of them shall be pricks in your eyes, and thorns in your sides, and shall vex you in the land wherein ye dwell. (Numbers 33:55).

Knowing his Scripture, Paul asks God to drive out the enemy who is troubling him. God answers that this particular enemy is there for a purpose and has to stay.

Therefore, it cannot be argued that Paul had a disease that God would not remove – it was a demon sent to humble him.

2. The man born blind.

> And as Jesus passed by, he saw a man which was blind from his birth. And his disciples asked him, saying, Master, who did sin, this man, or his parents, that he was born blind? Jesus answered, Neither hath this man sinned, nor his parents: but that the works of God should be made manifest in him. (John 9:1-3)

Aware of the link between sin and sickness as laid down in Deuteronomy, the Lord's disciples ask Him whether some specific sin of either the man or his parents has caused the blindness. In response, the Lord Jesus says that it is not the result of some specific sin *but in order that what God is doing in his life may be openly seen by everyone*. What was God doing in his life? Giving him his spiritual sight. How was this manifest? By the fact that his physical sight is given to him.

It is plain to see that the man was spiritually blind.

> Jesus heard that they had cast him out; and when he had found him, he said unto him, Dost thou believe on the Son of God? He answered and said, Who is he, Lord, that I might believe on him? (John 9:35-36)

Although he was more open to the Lord than all those around him, yet he hadn't received his spiritual sight. Therefore, the physical blindness was upon the man in demonstration of the fact that he was spiritually blind. The Lord Jesus heals him to pave the way for his spiritual eyes being opened.

> And Jesus said unto him, Thou hast both seen him, and it is he that talketh with thee. And he said, Lord, I believe. And he worshipped him. (John 9:35-38)

The Lord then confirms the link between his spiritual and physical condition:

> For judgment I am come into this world, that they which see not might see; and that they which see might be made blind. (John 9:39)

Though the sickness was not the result of sin, it was a demonstration that there was something amiss in the man's life: he was spiritually blind. Thus the man's body demonstrated what was happening in his spirit.

(For an exposition of the Book of Job, another place that might seem to contradict the doctrine, please see chapter 7, page 61).

Summary

Thus we see that throughout Scripture, the link between sickness and spiritual failing (or sin) is carefully taught and demonstrated.

Sickness entered the world with sin at the time of the Fall; in God's warnings to His people to keep the law, he makes it clear that failing to do so will lead to physical sickness; in numerous occasions throughout the Bible, sickness is given by God as a direct response to sin; in various cases, when people are healed, forgiveness of sin is linked with physical healing; finally at the cross, Christ's spiritual suffering for our sin was demonstrated by His physical suffering.

Moreover, those passages that might appear to contradict the doctrine, when actually examined fail to do so. Thus, we can say without a doubt that sickness in the body is always due to a failing in the spiritual life.

4

Sin and sickness – the purpose

If we are saying that God allows sickness to come on a person as a result of sin, we may ask, What is His purpose in doing this? For we must be certain that all things happen for a purpose.

> And we know that all things work together for good to them that love God, to them who are the called according to his purpose. (Romans 8:28)

Why, then, would a loving God allow His children to be ill? The answer is surely found in Hebrews 12:6, a passage that has a strong flavour of physical illness and healing.

> Whom the Lord loveth he chasteneth, and scourgeth every son whom he receiveth. (Hebrews 12:6)

We conclude, therefore, that sickness is sent by the Lord in order to correct us.

There is a principle in scripture that children should be corrected by corporal punishment.

> He that spareth his rod hateth his son: but he that loveth him chasteneth him betimes.
> Foolishness is bound in the heart of a child; but the rod of

correction shall drive it far from him.
Withhold not correction from the child: for if thou beatest
him with the rod, he shall not die. (Proverbs 13:24; 22:15;
23:13)

Therefore, it makes sense that the Lord should choose to correct
us with physical illness. This is not some act of harshness, but
the work of a loving God who always wants the best for His
children. Psalm 89, speaking specifically about the children of
Christ, i.e. New Testament believers, says that God will correct
them when they go astray.

If his children forsake my law, and walk not in my judgments;
if they break my statutes, and keep not my commandments;
then will I visit their transgression with the rod, and their
iniquity with stripes. Nevertheless my lovingkindness will I
not utterly take from him, nor suffer my faithfulness to fail.
(Psalm 89:30-33)

Rather than see us continue in sin, He takes steps to cause us to
turn from it. The desperation of the person's condition should
cause them to seek the face of God: when they do this, God
will reveal the cause of the illness and bring cleansing and
healing.

Careful chastisement

We must also conclude that when God is chastening us, He
is correcting us for something specific. When we looked at
the examples of sickness given to individuals in scripture,
we found that it was always the Lord's response to a specific
failing, not for general refining. What sort of father would
chastise His children for no reason? If our earthly parents
chastise us with a measure of justice and reason, according to
our specific misdemeanours, will not our heavenly Father be
infinitely more careful and precise in His dealings with us?

Furthermore we have had fathers of our flesh which corrected
us, and we gave them reverence: shall we not much rather

be in subjection unto the Father of spirits, and live? For they verily for a few days chastened us after their own pleasure; but he for our profit, that we might be partakers of his holiness. (Hebrews 12:9-10)

So the Lord gives illness in order to correct us, and He does so because it will have the desired effect upon us, if we respond to it properly, by submitting to God and seeking His face for the cause.

Therefore, chastening from the Lord should not be resisted, as if it were an attack of the Devil, but it should be responded to, by correcting our spiritual walk. Paul says to the Hebrews that chastening yields righteousness in those who respond to it, and the way to respond is to get the spiritual life sorted out. This, he says, will bring healing.

Now no chastening for the present seemeth to be joyous, but grievous: nevertheless afterward it yieldeth the peaceable fruit of righteousness unto them which are exercised thereby. Wherefore lift up the hands which hang down, and the feeble knees; And make straight paths for your feet, lest that which is lame be turned out of the way; but let it rather be healed. (Hebrews 12:11-13)

Here again, as we saw at times in the previous chapter, the physical and the spiritual is talked about interchangeably, as if they are two sides of the same issue.

Matthew 5:25 says:

Agree with thine adversary quickly, whiles thou art in the way with him; lest at any time the adversary deliver thee to the judge, and the judge deliver thee to the officer, and thou be cast into prison.

When the Lord steps into our lives as an adversary when we have started to go astray, we should respond quickly to Him.

5

Sin and sickness – the precision of the link

If we are to understand that the Lord chastens in response to specific sins, we may assume that the form of chastening will be appropriate and specific. In other words, that He corrects particular sins with particular sicknesses.

We might also assume that there would be a reason why a particular sickness was given in response to a particular sin.

His work is perfect: for all his ways are judgment: a God of truth and without iniquity, just and right is he. (Deuteronomy 32:4)

Would not a God who gives sickness in order to correct us use a form of illness that both highlights the nature of our problem and also helps us to deal with the problem? Let us see if this is the biblical pattern.

A. Leprosy

Let us look again at the story of King Uzziah in II Chronicles 26. His sin was to try to burn incense in the temple, and the reason why it was wrong was given by the priests:

It appertaineth not unto thee, Uzziah, to burn incense unto the LORD, but to the priests the sons of Aaron, that are consecrated to burn incense: go out of the sanctuary; for thou hast trespassed; neither shall it be for thine honor from the LORD God. (II Chronicles 26:18)

The sons of Aaron had been specially consecrated for the tasks of ministering in the sanctuary. Uzziah, as a common man and not a consecrated priest, was therefore 'unclean' for the purpose of offering incense, and his attempt to offer incense would have defiled the sanctuary.

The illness he received as a result was leprosy. Throughout the Bible, lepers are described as unclean. In Leviticus 13 and 14 it gives detailed instructions about leprosy, and again and again someone with leprosy is called 'unclean'.

The priest shall look on the plague in the skin of the flesh: and when the hair in the plague is turned white, and the plague in sight be deeper than the skin of his flesh, it is a plague of leprosy: and the priest shall look on him, and pronounce him unclean. (Leviticus 13:3).

Therefore, when Uzziah tried to offer incense, the Lord responded by smiting him with an illness that said 'You are unclean.' His sin might be summarised as 'presumption in taking a position with God not rightfully his,' or more simply, 'pride'.

In Numbers 12 we find two other characters committing this sin.

And Miriam and Aaron spake against Moses because of the Ethiopian woman whom he had married: for he had married an Ethiopian woman. And they said, Hath the LORD indeed spoken only by Moses? hath he not spoken also by us? And the LORD heard. (Numbers 12:1, 2)

So the Lord calls Miriam, Aaron and Moses into the tabernacle and says to Miriam and Aaron:

Hear now my words: If there be a prophet among you, I the LORD will make myself known unto him in a vision, and will speak unto him in a dream. My servant Moses is not so, who is faithful in all mine house. With him will I speak mouth to mouth, even apparently, and not in dark speeches; and the similitude of the LORD shall he behold: wherefore then were ye not afraid to speak against my servant Moses? And the anger of the LORD was kindled against them; and he departed. (Numbers 12:6-9)

Aaron and Miriam had suggested that they were in just the same position as Moses, that they had the same relationship with God. In response, God says that they were presumptuous, since Moses had been specially given a place of intimacy with Him. Note, therefore, the illness that Miriam receives:

And the cloud departed from off the tabernacle; and, behold, Miriam became leprous, white as snow: and Aaron looked upon Miriam, and, behold, she was leprous. (Numbers 12:10)

So we see that leprosy is twice given in response to the sin of presumption and pride. We observe too that there is a logical link between the illness and the sin.

Naaman was another character whose great stumbling-block was pride. When he came to Elisha for healing, and he was told to wash seven times in the Jordan, he was furious.

But Naaman was wroth, and went away, and said, Behold, I thought, He will surely come out to me, and stand, and call on the name of the LORD his God, and strike his hand over the place... Are not Abana and Pharpar, rivers of Damascus, better than all the waters of Israel? may I not wash in them, and be clean? So he turned and went away in a rage. And his servants came near, and spake unto him, and said, My father, if the prophet had bid thee do some great thing, wouldest thou not have done it? how much rather then, when he saith to thee, Wash, and be clean? (II Kings 5:11-13)

Naaman wants to believe that the rivers of his own country are as good as the Jordan. Like Uzziah and Miriam, his great notable sin is pride and presumption. The disease he has is leprosy. The moment he swallows his pride and obeys, he is healed.

> Then went he down, and dipped himself seven times in Jordan, according to the saying of the man of God: and his flesh came again like unto the flesh of a little child, and he was clean. (II Kings 5:14)

In the first two cases we saw that a particular illness was given in response to a particular sin; in this instance, however, we see that a specific illness is healed when a specific sin is dealt with.[7]

B. Haemorrhoids

When, in I Samuel 9, the Philistines took the Ark of the Covenant and brought it to Ashdod, the men were smitten with haemorrhoids. When the ark is moved to Gath, and then Ekron, the men in those cities are struck with the same disease. The same illness is given for the same sin.

Moreover, when we examine the sin, we can see why the Philistines received this particular disease. They had stolen the Ark of the Covenant, the place where the blood of atonement was poured out, and they had hidden it in a secret place. What is the disease they get?

> Emerods [bleeding veins] in their secret parts. (I Samuel 5:9)

There is a logical connection between the sin and the sickness. As we consider other examples, again we see that the illness given is appropriate for the sin.

---

[7] It will be observed that Gehazi, the servant of Elisha, was given leprosy after he ran after Naaman and, against his master's instructions, asked for a gift. Of course, Gehazi's most obvious sins in this regard are greed and lying. Yet the great underlying sin is still presumption, inasmuch as he decides that his judgement is better than Elisha's and takes it upon himself to reverse his decision. It is fitting, therefore, that he should receive Naaman's old disease.

C. Dumbness

If we look again at the story of Gabriel visiting Zacharias to foretell the birth of John the Baptist, we find that his sin is to doubt the words of the angel. He speaks out and says:

Whereby shall I know this? for I am an old man, and my wife well stricken in years.

In response to his inappropriate use of his voice, he loses it.

D. Withered hand

When Jeroboam stretches out his hand to lay hold of the man of God it is his hand that is smitten (I Kings 13).

Thus we see an initial scriptural indication that specific sicknesses are linked to specific sins and that there is a logical connection between them. But what is the practical evidence?

Practical evidence of the precise link between certain sins and sicknesses

After my healing from *candidiasis* I quickly came into contact with a number of other Christians with the same illness. I found that in every case the individuals strongly demonstrated that they had the same spiritual problem that I had had. I realised that by confessing the sin and getting right with God, they could be healed as I was.

I also started to consider other more minor ailments that I had, and to seek the Lord to find out their cause. As I did so, I found that any illness I got was the result of sin and could be dealt with by confessing it and turning from the sin.

In this way I have been delivered at various times from
- Acid reflux (bringing up the past)
- A bad back (carrying one's burdens)
- Colds (getting overheated with life and work)
- Constipation (lack of mercy)
- Various aches in arms and legs (various causes)
- Acne (pride/arrogance)

- Post nasal drip (contentiousness)
- Diarrhoea (wrong attitudes towards other Christians)

Moreover, as God has revealed to me the link between specific sins and sicknesses, I have found that everyone I speak to with a particular sickness quickly reveals in conversation the failing I have associated with it. This happens without any probing on my part. People with the same sickness are easily identifiable as having the same outstanding spiritual problem. For example, all people with a bad back carry their own burdens.

When I was seeking the Lord about other connections between sins and sickness, I thought about the great rise in cases of breast cancer. It seemed obvious to me that breast problems must relate to a mother's attitude towards her children since its anatomical purpose is to suckle children. I then thought of the great rise in abortions (terminations of pregnancy) in recent years and started to compare statistics. I found that, like for like, they produced the following astonishingly similar graphs.

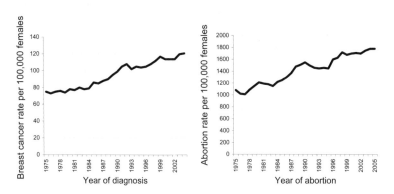

■ Age standardised breast cancer and abortion rates for England and Wales, 1975-2004/5.[8]

It is hard to miss the significance behind the matching graph lines. Interestingly, in the USA where abortion rates have been coming

---

[8] Source: Office for National Statistics

down, the age adjusted breast cancer rates have done the same.

How do we interpret the graphs then? Merely to say that though some women may show a bad attitude towards their children in ways other than having an abortion, when there is a national trend of not loving one's children, it will be demonstrated both in the rate of abortions and in the rate of breast cancer diagnoses. Moreover, there have been scientific studies that indicate that having an abortion increases the likelihood of contracting breast cancer.[9] Yet, a confession by the individuals involved of their sin in not loving their own children would bring forgiveness and physical healing.

The more the link between specific sins and sicknesses is investigated, the more obvious and undeniable the link appears to be.

The body as a picture of the soul

As we looked earlier at the Lord's death on the cross, we observed that the body could be seen as a picture of the soul, a demonstration in the physical of what is happening in the spiritual. Now as we start to observe the links between specific sins and sicknesses, we begin to find that each part of the body represents a different part of the spiritual life.

The more we look into the subject in the Bible, the more we find this to be the case. We have already seen that the physical and the spiritual are used interchangeably to describe the Lord's sufferings on the cross. However, if we look closely, we find that this is the case throughout the Bible.

We are fully familiar with certain parts of the body being used as pictures of the soul. The Bible speaks of the 'pure in heart', and conversely of being 'stiff necked'. Those who use the Authorized Version will be familiar with phrases such as 'bowels

---

[9] For example, a study by Janet Daling found the following: 'Among women who had been pregnant at least once, the risk of breast cancer in those who had experienced an induced abortion was 50% higher than among other women'. Journal of the National Cancer Institute, Vol. 86, No. 21, 1584-1592, November 2, 1994 © 1994 Oxford University Press

of compassion' (1 John 3:17), which is an accurate translation of the Greek original. However, we may be surprised to discover that every time the Bible uses the word 'reins' (that is, like the reins of a horse, the thing by which we are guided) in both the Old Testament and New, the word used is 'kidneys'.[10]

Equally, in various places in the Bible it refers to an illness brought about by sin as being incurable. An example is given in Jeremiah 30.

> For thus saith the LORD, Thy bruise is incurable, and thy wound is grievous. (Jeremiah 30:12).

However, the word translated 'incurable' also means desperately wicked and is translated this way in Jeremiah 17.

> The heart is deceitful above all things, and desperately wicked: who can know it? (Jeremiah 17:9)

So we see the above verse could be translated 'the heart is incurable' or 'the will is desperately wicked'. Again, the physical and the spiritual are used interchangeably.

The mass of information
As we search through the Bible we find there is a mass of information about different parts of the body and their spiritual meaning, and in each case the connection is logical. Thus God has provided us with numerous indications in His Word of the causes of specific illnesses, as shown in Section Two, and we do well to observe them. The more we really examine these scriptures, the more concrete the link between sin and sickness seems to be.

---

[10] It is important for this reason to use an accurate translation of the Bible. The Authorised (King James) Version remains the most accurate, because, more than any other version, it simply translates what the original text says, without adding its own slant or interpretation.

6

The doctrine in detail

We come, therefore, to the place where we have established from the Bible the following points:

- There is a link between sin and sickness.
- Sickness is God's way of showing us that there is some failing in our lives.
- There is a link between specific sins and specific sicknesses.

Therefore all sickness is an indication of something that needs correcting in our spiritual lives. The nature and location of the illness will help to indicate the nature of the sin. Once the sin is identified, it can be confessed and abandoned, and the healing can come easily.

Entire provision has been made for our physical healing by the Lord Jesus in the work of the cross. Just as in His death he paid the price for our sin, in suffering physically the Lord Jesus paid for our physical healing. Not only did He carry our sin, but He bore our physical suffering too.

Surely he hath borne our griefs [literally, *diseases*], and carried our sorrows [or *pains*]: yet we did esteem him

stricken, smitten of God, and afflicted. But he was wounded
for our transgressions, he was bruised for our iniquities:
the chastisement of our peace was upon him; and **with his
stripes we are healed**. (Isaiah 53:5)

Who his own self bare our sins in his own body on the tree,
that we, being dead to sins, should live unto righteousness: **by
whose stripes ye were healed.** (I Peter 2:24)

If we allow some sin to remain in our lives subsequent to
conversion, the Lord, in order to correct us, may allow part of our
bodies to become ill. Once the sin is dealt with, healing comes
instantly.

In the case of the unregenerate man, in some cases their illness
may point to the very fact that they are unsaved (such as blindness
showing that they are spiritually blind – Isaiah 35:4-6). However
they may have other illnesses relating to individual sins that will
not be healed until those sins are dealt with.

It is also very important to understand that illness is given
by God as loving correction. Therefore, he deals with us as
individuals. Consequently,

- Just because a person commits a sin, it doesn't mean they
  will necessarily become ill. God will correct a person at a
  time and in a manner that is appropriate for them. However,
  we can safely say that anyone who has the illness commits
  the appropriate sin, because God does not correct for no
  purpose.
- Just because God is correcting a person, it does not mean
  that they are worse than other people on that issue; it just
  means they are not as good as God wants them to be.
  For example, a person's ministry may involve caring for
  people. Now they may be far more loving than most people
  anyway. Yet, because this attribute is so important for them
  as an individual, God may set a higher standard for them.
  Consequently, if they are not as loving as He wants them to
  be, he may allow them to become ill. Thus we see old saints
  who have heard the Lord's voice for many years becoming

deaf in old age: it is not that they are necessarily worse than others at listening to God, but that God says that they are not as good as He wants them to be.

Let us look at the doctrine in further detail by answering some important questions.

Is all sickness a result of specific sin?

We believe that all sickness is indicative of a specific spiritual situation that needs correcting and in most cases we would term this sin.

As in the case of the man born blind (*see page 29*), it can mean simply that a person is unsaved, is spiritually blind. But all sickness means a spiritual failing of some kind.

Why am I ill? Is God angry and punishing me?

No, God is not angry and is not punishing you. God gives us illness in order to correct us. He does it out of love. He sees some spiritual problem, some sin, and He wants to set us free from that. He may use various means to correct us, such as preaching, and advice from other people. However, we are often so blind to our sins that we don't see them. So He gives us a physical illness to try to wake us up to the fact that we have some sin that has not been dealt with. This should force us to humble ourselves and seek Him so that He can reveal what is wrong.

Since the Lord gives illness in order to correct us, and He corrects those He loves, it is often people who are really seeking to go on with God who fall ill.

Does sin always show itself as sickness?

No, not always.

This is explained when Paul gives Timothy advice about alleviating his particular symptoms.

Drink no longer water, but use a little wine for thy stomach's sake and thine often infirmities. Some men's sins are open beforehand, going before to judgment; and some men they follow after. (I Timothy 5:23-24)

He explains that some men's sins are openly displayed by sickness, but that for others the consequences come later. In Timothy's case, the particular sin problem that he had was manifest in his stomach problems and other illnesses.

Why does God choose to correct some people this way and not others?

Since illness is given to us as correction, God gives the illness because he has deemed it really important that we are corrected on that issue. Someone who is a pastor needs to be good at listening. If they don't listen well enough to people, they may become ill (in this case, become deaf) because it is so important that they are corrected. However, someone else may also be a poor listener, but that is not their chief problem, so the Lord isn't dealing with that at the moment. Perhaps their main problem is that they have a harsh tongue and so they may be suffering mouth problems.

We may also look at Christians who are terribly nice but not terribly spiritual and wonder why they enjoy such good health. In reply to this we would say that those who have been given more potential by the Lord are corrected more firmly.

For unto whomsoever much is given, of him shall be much required: and to whom men have committed much, of him they will ask the more. (Luke 12:48)

We need to remember that each illness is a loving act of correction. God has given the illness because it is very important that the individual is right on that particular issue.

Why does God use sickness rather than another means?

Because it is the most effective. There is surely nothing we hate so much as physical pain, so it causes us to come to our senses, to start being serious with God and begin to seek Him.

In addition to this, each illness is corrective in its own right. For example, someone who doesn't listen to other people will receive deafness as a result. This causes them to ask people to repeat things that they have not heard, and they end up straining to hear so hard that they listen and take it in as well. In some cases, they will be so deaf that things will need to be written down. This will make it even more certain that they will pay attention to what is being said.

Can all sickness be healed this way?
Yes, absolutely.

Inasmuch as sickness is simply a consequence of our sin, and since Christ has died to save us from our sins and suffered to deliver us from sickness, He desires that everyone should be healed. When we are cleansed from sin we are delivered from sickness. Nowhere in scripture does it say that sickness is to be accepted and lived with. Christians are to expect afflictions, persecutions and difficulties: but sickness has been fully paid for by Christ at the cross and should be dealt with.

It is interesting to note in James 5:13-14 that he says that if anyone is afflicted, he should pray (presumably for grace to endure), but that if anyone is sick, that he should call for the elders of the church in order that he might be healed.

What about going to the doctor?
I believe that the Lord is saddened when we go to earthly doctors with their limited knowledge, receiving drugs which further damage our bodies,[11] when we could go to the Great Physician and receive our perfect healing and at the same time have our spiritual problem dealt with as well.

If God in His wisdom has given us an illness in order to teach us something spiritual, if we seek to get rid of the illness without dealing with the sin it defeats the object of God's giving us the

---

[11] The World Health Organisation says: 'All medicines have side effects and some of those can be damaging. The effects of any medical intervention cannot be predicted with absolute certainty. No drug is totally devoid of risk.' Fact sheet N°293. September 2005

sickness in the first place. It is like trying to shut our ears to God.

The lesson from scripture is clearly that we should go to the Lord, not to earthly physicians. We find this to be taught in the life of King Asa.

> And Asa in the thirty and ninth year of his reign was diseased in his feet, until his disease was exceeding great: yet in his disease he sought not to the LORD, but to the physicians. (II Chronicles 16:12)

Consequently he was not healed. The lesson is also found in the story of the woman with the issue of blood.

> And a certain woman, which had an issue of blood twelve years, And had suffered many things of many physicians, and had spent all that she had, and was nothing bettered, but rather grew worse, When she had heard of Jesus, came in the press behind, and touched his garment. For she said, If I may touch but his clothes, I shall be whole. And straightway the fountain of her blood was dried up; and she felt in her body that she was healed of that plague. (Mark 5:25-29)

It seems clear that the Lord wants us to go to Him rather than to human doctors.

There is a difference, however, between nursing and medicine. If, for example, a person has a serious wound, it would be wise to have it bathed and bandaged at a hospital. If a person has a fever, they should obviously be looked after. Yet in this situation, the Lord wants us to seek to Him for healing, not to the doctors. For this reason, there is no reason to receive medicine and surgery. When a sick person seeks the Lord, he will find that his symptoms recede, enabling him to feel well enough to meet with God.

A number of times in the Bible it describes a person's illness as being incurable:

> For thus saith the LORD, Thy bruise is incurable, and thy wound is grievous. (Jeremiah 30:12. See also Micah 1:9; Nahum 3:19; 2 Chronicles 21:18; Job 34:6; Jeremiah 15:18; Jeremiah 30:15)

What is interesting about many of the illnesses that Christians get is that they are incurable, thus they are forced to seek the Lord, rather than go to the doctor. Christians will also often find that their appointments with the doctor are cancelled again and again, as the Lord gives them repeated opportunities to go to Him instead. How much better for us to go to the Lord in every circumstance.

A note of caution, however. To go neither to the Lord, nor to a human doctor is not an option. Moreover, if a person is currently taking a course of medication, they should not stop taking it unless they are clear from the Lord that it is right for them to do so. When the Lord speaks, His word comes to the believer with a sense of peace. To stop taking drugs without dealing with the underlying spiritual problem could be an act of presumption, with serious consequences. When a person is healed, they are sure of it, and continuing to take the medication will not alter this. Avoid the temptation to 'show your faith' by ceasing to take medication. To stop taking medication is not an act of faith in itself.

(Please see also Appendix 1: What about Doctors *by Harold Horton, page 89).*

I know the physical cause of my illness. Doesn't this disprove the doctrine?

Very often we will identify an original physical cause of our illness: 'I've had leg problems ever since I injured it playing hockey 3 years ago'; 'I've had bowel problems ever since eating a takeaway a year ago'.

There will always be some physical element that starts our illness, but that physical factor has been allowed by God.

> Who hath made man's mouth? or who maketh the dumb, or deaf, or the seeing, or the blind? have not I the LORD? (Exodus 4:11)

If there had been no sin, God's hand of Grace would not have been removed and we would not have been injured or fallen ill.

What about injury as opposed to sickness?

Injury falls into the same category as illness. When we are injured, it is because God has allowed it to happen, and it will indicate something amiss in our spiritual life. If there were nothing wrong, we could not have been injured.

To give an example, I used to be slightly interested in shooting. I didn't do much of it, but one day, I thought I would renew my interest, as a way of recreation and rest. I got my gun out and started cleaning it. Within a very short time I had seriously damaged my thumb, slicing the end of it almost off. I later realised that God was telling me that shooting would distract me from my work, and that I shouldn't touch it. Now, if I ever think about shooting again, the scar on my thumb starts to throb.

The only exception to this rule would appear to be sufferings from persecution. There is a privilege in suffering for the Lord, and this is the one and only type of physical suffering that is for His glory (Acts 5:41; Acts 9:16; Colossians 1:24).

Various people were left sick in the Bible. Why were they not healed?

When the Lord gives an illness in response to sin, it may take the individual a long time to see their sin and to confess it. The sickness itself is remedial, in that it helps the sufferer to deal with their sin. So when someone is ill, even a great man of God cannot necessarily bring the person through to healing immediately.

Therefore, it is not surprising that Paul says:

Trophimus have I left at Miletum sick. (II Timothy 4:20)

In the same way he advises Timothy to arrange his diet to alleviate his illness.

Drink no longer water, but use a little wine for thy stomach's sake and thine often infirmities. (I Timothy 5:23)

This is in spite of the fact, as we have already seen, that Paul indicates that Timothy's illness is a result of sin *(see page 44)*.

Another example of someone remaining ill in the New Testament is Epaphroditus.

For indeed he was sick nigh unto death: but God had mercy
on him; and not on him only, but on me also, lest I should have
sorrow upon sorrow. Because for the work of Christ he was
nigh unto death, not regarding his life, to supply your lack of
service toward me. (Philippians 2:27, 30)

It seems that Epaphroditus had become ill through overwork,
in attempting to fill the shortfall left by the Philippians' lack of
service. It is not surprising that he would fall ill, since overwork
is a sin. The Lord never gives us too much work to do. If our
brother doesn't do his particular task in the Kingdom of God,
we should not feel it is down to us to take it on ourselves. Doing
that may cause us to do our own work badly. Far better to correct
the brother.

Robert Murray M'Cheyne once said of his own overwork,
'God gave me a horse and a message. I have killed the horse,
and I can no longer deliver the message.'

Should we not expect our bodies to waste away as we grow old?

As we grow older, we seem to get more and more physical
ailments. We might suppose that this is merely part of old age
and has nothing to do with sin. The issue, however, has to do
with strength.

In I John 2, the Apostle indicates a difference between the
spiritual experiences of different age groups. He says,

I have written unto you, fathers, because ye have known him
that is from the beginning. I have written unto you, young men,
because ye are strong, and the word of God abideth in you,
and ye have overcome the wicked one. (I John 2:14)

His statement seems to refer both to spiritual age and physical
age, but he makes it clear that one of the marks of youth is
strength. Godly young men, we often find, have huge amounts
of zeal and strength, and they press through to God. Their
discernment can be very sharp and they can be very sensitive to
hear the Lord's voice. Because everything is new and fresh, they

have the spiritual energy to overcome the devil (v. 13), be strong in dealing with sin, and to go on quickly with God. What they lack, however, is wisdom and a long term knowledge of God.

Older Christians, however, have the greater knowledge of God which comes from a long walk with Him, and they may know greater depths of devotion to Him, yet they have less strength and zeal. Consequently, some of their spiritual faculties may decline. It is interesting to note that very often one faculty may decline but another remains sharp.

An example of this is the prophet Ahijah. In I Kings 14, we are told that Jeroboam sends his wife in disguise to speak to Ahijah. However, it says that 'Ahijah could not see; for his eyes were set by reason of his age' (I Kings 14:4). Because Ahijah could not see, the Lord says to him,

> Behold, the wife of Jeroboam cometh to ask a thing of thee for her son; for he is sick: thus and thus shalt thou say unto her: for it shall be, when she cometh in, that she shall feign herself to be another woman. (I Kings 14:5)

Now the word used for 'see' also means 'to discern'. Thus it says that Ahijah could neither see physically nor discern, and he would have been unable to tell that the woman was Jeroboam's wife come in disguise. However, his spiritual hearing is still excellent, so God speaks to him instead. The ensuing story shows that his physical hearing was just as good.

> And it was so, when Ahijah heard the sound of her feet, as she came in at the door, that he said, Come in, thou wife of Jeroboam. (I Kings 14:6)

Similarly, we may think of Fanny Crosby, the great hymn-writer, who was blind from early childhood. She was obviously a tremendously spiritual person, and could hear God's voice and knew His heart. Yet this does not mean she could not have been lacking in the area of spiritual discernment. Very often, people who have lost one sense, such as sight, say that other senses become much more sensitive as a result. So we may understand that Crosby's other spiritual senses were heightened as a result of her lack in this one area.

However, if we realise that a faculty is failing, there is no reason why we should not confess it to the Lord and receive healing. The Bible says,

> Bless the LORD, O my soul, and forget not all his benefits: Who satisfieth thy mouth with good things; so that thy youth is renewed like the eagle's. (Psalm 103:2, 5)

With regard to physical strength, the Bible says that God gives us strength to do just what he wants us to do.

> As thy days, so shall thy strength be. (Deuteronomy 33:25)

Therefore, we will have enough strength to do what we are called to do but not necessarily what we want to do. As we grow older, the Lord may call us to spend most of our time in prayer, to be like Moses, with young Joshuas going into battle. I think very often He does. You do not require much physical strength for prayer; in fact, you are better being weak. However, if in old age we try to do the work of the young, to be a Joshua instead of a Moses, we will feel we don't have enough strength. Therefore, in old age, we can be perfectly fit and well, and have just the right amount of energy for what we are called to do.

Some may argue that Paul speaks of the outward man perishing, and that this indicates a gradual wearing away of the body. Paul does indeed say,

> For which cause we faint not; but though our outward man perish, yet the inward man is renewed day by day. (II Corinthians 4:16)

However, the context of the verse is clearly the persecutions which they were enduring, which included physical suffering:

> But we have this treasure in earthen vessels, that the excellency of the power may be of God, and not of us. We are troubled on every side, yet not distressed; we are perplexed, but not in despair; persecuted, but not forsaken; cast down, but not destroyed; always bearing about in the body the dying of the

Lord Jesus, that the life also of Jesus might be made manifest in our body. (II Corinthians 4:7-10)

What about children?

A child is by nature a sinner from the moment of conception. David says,

Behold, I was shapen in iniquity; and in sin did my mother conceive me. (Psalm 51:5)

Again, the apostle Paul speaks of how we have all inherited Adam's sinful nature.

By the offence of one judgment came upon all men to condemnation.
By one man's disobedience many were made sinners. (Romans 5:18, 19)

Consequently, all children are born sinners and will sin as soon as they are born: it is what they naturally do. Therefore God will use sickness to highlight and correct sin, or a particular sinful disposition, in a child just as in an adult. This should be seen as an alarm bell to the parents, to show them there is something wrong in the life of the child.

This applies to babies as it does to older children. We may find this surprising, but we should remember that John the Baptist was filled with the Holy Spirit even in the womb and had his own response to God even then (Luke 1:15, 41). Though a baby is physically and mentally undeveloped, it has a spirit which is presumably fully mature from the start of life[12], can relate to God, and therefore is able to sin.[13]

The first step when seeking healing for a sick child can always

---

[12] In the case of the Lord Jesus, though he was born with the usual physical and presumably verbal limitations of infancy, yet he was spiritually perfect and unchanging.

[13] Augustine said, 'The infant's innocence lies in the weakness of his body and not in the infant mind. I have myself observed a baby to be jealous, though it could not speak; it was livid as it watched another infant at the breast'. (Confessions 1:VII:11)

be simply to pray for his healing. The Lord may graciously intervene, working in the child's spirit and delivering him from the spiritual problem as well as the physical ailment. *(See also* The role of Elders, *p.71)*. However, when healing does not come, it will be necessary to seek the Lord for the spiritual cause of the illness. When the cause has been discovered, those ministering to the child can respond by praying for his deliverance from the sin issue, helping him to recognise and turn from the sin, and dealing with any issues in their own lives which may be affecting the child.

For example, if a child has tonsil problems, this is because he doesn't have a healthy conscience about what he is saying and thinking. The parents therefore need to show the child what he is doing wrong so that he can confess it to God and turn from it. The child can then be prayed for and receive his healing. The parents can also educate him in being careful about what he says, to think before speaking and to say things that will please God. They can also correct and chastise the child when he commits the particular sin.

In the case of babies, when healing does not come, the parents should seek to know the cause of the illness and having discovered it, respond by helping the child accordingly and praying for its healing. For example, if a baby has a cold, it will indicate that it is restless. The parents should find ways of helping and teaching the baby to rest. They can then pray for the child and it will be healed.

It should also be noted that children of any age are affected and influenced by the spiritual state and behaviour of those around them. Even though they may not yet understand words, they are still communing with people. We see this in the way babies respond to the moods of those they are with. Therefore, any sinful attitude in the parents may influence a child. For example, a child who has received a cold because of restlessness could have been affected by either restlessness in its parents, or by their not allowing it proper opportunity to rest. When a child is ill, therefore, the parents should seek the Lord to discover whether they are sinning in an area that has influenced the child, causing it to be ill. (*For more on babies, see also* Congenital Illnesses *below)*.

What about children with congenital illnesses?
When a parent has a particular sinful disposition, the child will

very often inherit it. Therefore, when a child is born into such circumstances that it is certain to grow up with a particular sin problem, the Lord will sometimes take preventative measures and give the child an illness. For example, a child is born to a woman with HIV. Let's say she contracted the disease from promiscuity and has a weak conscience. If nothing is done to prevent it, the child will grow up to be promiscuous just like its mother: everything it sees in its home life and everything in its own natural disposition will ensure this. The child is therefore born with HIV itself in order to try to stop this happening. If the mother sees her sin and turns from it, she will be in a position to bring the child up in the right way, thus preventing it from committing the same sin. Through faith in Christ she can be cleansed from her own sin, and then she can pray for the child to be healed as well.

Obviously, the significance of this doctrine can be seen in societies where promiscuity is rife. When a whole generation has turned from God and sexual license is the norm, a disease such as HIV may be given to cause people to wake up and turn from their sin.

When nothing is being done to prevent a child growing up with a particular sin problem, when the parents do not respond to the sickness by turning from their sin, God may allow the child to die as the final means of preventing the degeneracy within the family.

To give another example, two Christian parents are very gifted intellectually. This has caused them to go through life trusting in their own intellect rather than God, and so it has had a very limiting effect on their spiritual lives. In order to prevent this problem being repeated in the next generation, the Lord may allow their children to be born with learning difficulties. This will ensure the child is free from this particular sin, and it may have a corrective humbling effect on the parents. If the parents were to recognize the problem and turn from their sin, they could pray for the child and it would be healed. However, the illness has a remedial effect in its own right.

It must be noted, however, that a child does not suffer for the sins of its parents, but rather inherits their sinful disposition. It is therefore born with its own sinful attitude, and this is what God may seek to correct with disease.

Some may argue that children cannot be affected by the sins of the parents, yet the Bible and everyday evidence both teach us that they can. The Bible teaches that children are 'in the loins' of their parents.[14] For this reason, all the descendents of Adam inherited his sinful nature.[15] Similarly, in practical terms, if two people commit incest, any ill effects the child may suffer will be the direct result of the parents' sin. It is clear that children *are* affected by the sins of their parents. However, although they may inherit certain dispositions from their parents, they are only responsible before God for the sins that they commit themselves. Thus we see, when God speaks about visiting sins of parents upon their children, it only applies when the children continue in rebellion against God.[16]

> I the LORD thy God am a jealous God, visiting the iniquity of the fathers upon the children unto the third and fourth generation **of them that hate me**. (Exodus 20:5)

We see this in the case of David. In response to his sin in committing adultery with Bathsheba and killing Uriah (II Samuel 11) the Lord says, 'the sword shall never depart from thine house'. Consequently, Ammon, Absalom and Adonijah all die by the sword, but their own lives were marked by exceptional wickedness.

Ezekiel 18 is one of the passages that deal with this subject. In this chapter, the Jews are complaining that their captivity is a result of their parents' sins. They have been saying, 'The fathers

---

[14] Hebrews 7:9   [15] Romans 5:19

[16] Some people would teach that, as we are affected by the sins of our ancestors, we should therefore seek out the sins of our forebears in order to break free from the effects. This is quite unscriptural. Although the sins of our ancestors do have an effect on us naturally, when we are born again we are free from all this: 'Therefore if any man be in Christ, he is a new creature: old things are passed away; behold, all things are become new' (II Cor. 5:17). We are no longer in Adam but in Christ (I Cor. 15:22). After the new birth, the only things that affect us are our own fleshly attitudes (which are dealt with by putting the old nature to death) and our personal sins from day to day, which can be dealt with by confession (I John 1:9).

have eaten sour grapes, and the children's teeth are set on edge.' But God responds by saying,

> The soul that sinneth, it shall die. The son shall not bear the iniquity of the father, neither shall the father bear the iniquity of the son: the righteousness of the righteous shall be upon him, and the wickedness of the wicked shall be upon him. But if the wicked will turn from all his sins that he hath committed, and keep all my statutes, and do that which is lawful and right, he shall surely live, he shall not die. (Ezekiel 18:19-21)

The Lord is establishing a point concerning spiritual death. Children will not die spiritually for the sins of the parents and vice versa. [Spiritual death, or the death of the soul, means eternal death, eternity in hell. It is clear from verses 25-32 that that is the meaning of the passage.]

However, in the case of the Jews, the sins of their parents have caused them to be born into captivity. That captivity is God's loud-hailer to the nation, waking them up to the fact that they have been committing idolatry. The fact that the children remain in captivity is an indication that they are repeating the sins of their parents: if they repent and turn from their sins, their captivity will be ended. Although the children have been born into captivity, their eternal destiny is not decided by that, but by their own obedience to God. Nonetheless, the captivity should serve as a warning to the children not to continue in their parents' sins but to repent and turn back to God.

> Cast away from you all your transgressions, whereby ye have transgressed; and make you a new heart and a new spirit: for why will ye die, O house of Israel? (Ezekiel 18:31)

The same thing is true in the case of physical illness brought about as a result of sin. By inheriting its parents' sinful disposition, a child may be born ill. That does not affect the eternal destiny of the child – it is only responsible for its own sins. Rather, it is a trumpet call to both the parents and the child as it grows up that something is wrong. Without it, the sins of the parents are likely to be repeated by generation after generation. It is a fact of everyday life that children are apt to repeat the sins of the parents. So the illness is given to the child to prevent it from following in the sins of the parents: it is an act of grace on the part of God to prevent degeneracy. If the parents do not see their own sin, they will continue to bring up their child in a way that encourages or permits that same sin. (*See also* <u>Congenital Disorders</u>).

The proper way to respond, therefore, is to realize that the illness is allowed by God for a purpose, and for the parents to confess their sins and repent.

If a parent confesses the sin and gets right with God and is able then to bring up the child in a way that counters this problem, they can pray for the child and he can be healed.

If a child is old enough to, he can confess his own sinful disposition that has caused the illness and be freed from the disease. It will obviously be a natural part of their confession for them to acknowledge before God that it has been a family trait.

And they that are left of you shall pine away in their iniquity in your enemies' lands; and also in the iniquities of their fathers shall they pine away with them. If they shall confess their iniquity, and the iniquity of their fathers, with their trespass which they trespassed against me, and that also they have walked contrary unto me; and that I also have walked contrary unto them, and have brought them into the land of their enemies; if then their uncircumcised hearts be humbled, and they then accept of the punishment of their iniquity: then will I remember my covenant with Jacob, and also my covenant with Isaac, and also my covenant with Abraham will I remember; and I will remember the land. (Leviticus 26:39-42)

In cases where a child is being cared for by others, a third party Christian may pray for the child, acknowledging the sin issue concerned, and the child will be healed. Since the illness is given to prevent the child growing up to sin in this area, a guardian who knows the problem and acknowledges it before God can be careful to bring the child up in a way that prevents it from perpetuating this sinful trait.

How can unbelievers be helped?

Sickness in unbelievers is caused by sin, just as in believers. Therefore, in order for them to be healed, they need to be cleansed from their sin. Obviously, the first thing is for them to be born again.

They may have an illness which is linked to the fact that they are unsaved. For example, someone may have physical blindness to demonstrate their spiritual blindness. When they recognize their spiritual blindness, confess it, and trust in Christ, they will receive their physical sight. (Blindness remaining after being born again would indicate there was still an issue causing spiritual blindness that had not been resolved. This would not affect the person's salvation).

They may, however, have a sickness that is just the result of a particular sin. Obviously, in order to be cleansed from this as well as all their other sins, they need to be born again. The sin that the sickness reveals may be a good starting point for them to recognize their sin in general.

It is possible, though, that someone can be born again, but have a deep-rooted sin that is not dealt with at salvation. They may in consequence retain a sickness relating to that sin. For example, a man may be continually bringing up the past, bemoaning the things he has suffered. As a result of this he has acid reflux. He comes to Christ and is saved, but retains the sin and the sickness. The sickness will not be dealt with until the individual sin is recognized and confessed.

Why, in scripture and modern-day experience, are some people miraculously healed without reference to sin?

In certain circumstances, the Lord may choose to heal someone to pave the way for repentance. Paul says to the Romans,

> The goodness of God leadeth thee to repentance. (Romans 2:4)

God will therefore sometimes do a work of grace in someone, to encourage them to turn to Him. We see this in the case of the man born blind, who received his physical sight first and then his spiritual sight. The Bible calls healings of this kind 'gifts of healing' (I Corinthians 12:9, 28, 30) – they are free gifts, coming entirely by the grace of God and not dependent upon the one receiving the healing. They happen simply to show the goodness and greatness of God and to cause the person to turn to Him. In such circumstances it is to be expected that the person will repent as a result of the healing. To one man that Jesus healed, He said,

> Behold, thou art made whole: sin no more, lest a worse thing come unto thee. (John 5:14)

This indicates that the man had received a healing and was expected as a result to turn from his sin. It also indicates that a person who is healed may fall ill again if they return to the sin.

On some occasions, a person may turn from their sin at the moment they are healed by the working of the Holy Spirit, but not see the relationship between the two or be fully conscious of what has happened. Thus healing will very often accompany the preaching of the gospel (Mark 16:20).

In normal circumstances, when God has given an illness to a believer, it is because there is a deep-rooted sin in that person's life that needs drastic action. They will almost certainly be unaware of the sin, so giving them a gift of healing would mean that the sin was never dealt with.

If God heals me and I fall into the sin again, will I become ill again?

Yes. Jesus said to the impotent man,

> Behold, thou art made whole: sin no more, lest a worse thing come unto thee. (John 5:14)

The doctrine of sin and sickness continues to apply after healing has been received.

For further questions from Scripture, please see Appendix 4, *page 104.*

7

My Servant Job
(Why men of God fall ill)

One of the things that will puzzle many people about this doctrine is the fact that men of God fall ill, sometimes while quite young, and even die from the disease. A useful study in this regard is Job.

An overview of the book of Job
At the start of the book of Job we are given a description of Job by the Lord:

> Hast thou considered my servant Job, that there is none like him in the earth, a perfect and an upright man, one that feareth God, and escheweth evil? (Job 1:8)

Satan is then allowed to test Job, to see whether his devotion to God is simply due to his prosperous circumstances. Satan destroys his children, his livestock and his servants. He then smites Job with 'sore boils from the sole of his foot unto his crown' (Job 2:7).

Most of the book of Job consists of Job expostulating with God, his three friends maintaining that Job's suffering is God's judgement upon sin, and Job asserting his integrity.

The book finishes with God reproving Job for arguing with Him and challenging him to acknowledge his human limitations and frailty before God. God also reproves his friends for misrepresenting Him to Job. Job is commended for his correct view of God.

Perhaps the most helpful part of the book in seeking to gain a true interpretation of what is going on is the judgement given by Elihu. He is not one of Job's three friends, but a young man who clearly speaks for God.

> Then was kindled the wrath of Elihu the son of Barachel the Buzite, of the kindred of Ram: against Job was his wrath kindled, because he justified himself rather than God. Also against his three friends was his wrath kindled, because they had found no answer, and yet had condemned Job. (Job 32:2, 3)

He begins by reproving Job's friends for simply condemning Job without having an answer to his situation.

> Behold, I waited for your words; I gave ear to your reasons, whilst ye searched out what to say. Yea, I attended unto you, and, behold, there was none of you that convinced Job, or that answered his words: (Job 32:11, 12)

He then goes on to do for Job what they had failed to do – give a solution to his problems. He shows that God gives sickness in order to chasten and correct: it is one of Gods ways of speaking to man when other means fail.

> For God speaketh once, yea twice, yet man perceiveth it not... He is chastened also with pain upon his bed, and the multitude of his bones with strong pain: so that his life abhorreth bread, and his soul dainty meat. His flesh is consumed away, that it cannot be seen; and his bones that were not seen stick out. (Job 33:14, 18-21)

In trying to get through to a man, God may even take him to the point of death.

> Yea, his soul draweth near unto the grave, and his life to the destroyers. (Job 33:22)

However, if someone is able to point out to the man his error so that he can repent, then God will forgive him and heal his body.

> If there be a messenger with him, an interpreter, one among a thousand, to shew unto man his uprightness [or *what is right for him (ASV)*]: then he is gracious unto him, and saith, Deliver him from going down to the pit: I have found a ransom. His flesh shall be fresher than a child's: he shall return to the days of his youth: he shall pray unto God, and he will be favourable unto him: and he shall see his face with joy: for he will render unto man his righteousness. He looketh upon men, and if any say, I have sinned, and perverted that which was right, and it profited me not; he will deliver his soul from going into the pit, and his life shall see the light. Lo, all these things worketh God oftentimes with man, to bring back his soul from the pit, to be enlightened with the light of the living. (Job 33:30)

Elihu goes on to say that Job has been wrong to charge God with injustice. Job has asserted his own righteousness, and claimed that it is therefore unfair for God to allow him to suffer:

> For Job hath said, I am righteous: and God hath taken away my judgment. Should I lie against my right? my wound is incurable without transgression. (Job 34:6)

Job says that God has given him an incurable wound for no reason: why should he lie and say that he has sinned when he hasn't? In response, Elihu says that God is just and gives to men what is appropriate:

> Therefore hearken unto me ye men of understanding: far be it from God, that he should do wickedness; and from the Almighty, that he should commit iniquity. For the work of a man shall he render unto him, and cause every man to find according to his ways. Yea, surely God will not do wickedly, neither will the Almighty pervert judgment. (Job 34:10-12)

He also gives Job a clear example of how, in his illness, he should respond to God:

> Surely it is meet to be said unto God, I have borne chastisement, I will not offend any more: that which I see not teach thou me: if I have done iniquity, I will do no more. (Job 34:1)

After Elihu has finished speaking, God speaks directly to Job, confirming much of what Elihu has said, and reproving Job for his arrogance.

A perfect heart

In order to understand the main lesson of this book we need to return to God's original commendation of Job as a 'perfect' man.

What does God mean when he describes Job as perfect? He certainly does not mean he is sinless, for 'all have sinned, and come short of the glory of God' (Romans 3:23). Rather, he means that Job had a heart that always wanted to please the Lord. David Wilkerson, in his book *Hungry for More of Jesus,* describes what it means to have a perfect heart:

> To come to grips with the idea of perfection, we first must understand that perfection does not mean a sinless, flawless existence. People judge by outward appearances, by what they see. But God judges the heart, the unseen motives (1 Samuel 16:7). David had a perfect heart toward God 'all the days of his life' – yet David failed the Lord often. In fact, his life was marked forever by adultery and a notorious murder.
>
> No, perfection in the Lord's eyes means something entirely different. ...It means to finish what has been started, to make a complete performance. John Wesley called this concept of perfection 'constant obedience'; that is, a perfect heart is a responsive heart, one that answers quickly and totally all the Lord's wooings, whisperings and warnings. Such a heart says at all times, 'Speak, Lord, for Your servant is listening. Show me the path, and I will walk in it.'[17]

Therefore, in saying that Job was perfect, God was not saying that he was sinless, but rather that He always sought to do what was right. We see this in the fact that, at the beginning of the book, Job

---

[17] *Hungry for More of Jesus*, (Rickfords Hill Publishing, 2003), p. 46.

offers burnt offerings 'continually' on behalf of his children just in case they have sinned (Job 1:5).

However, there was still in Job a sinful attitude that needed dealing with, namely an arrogance before God of which he was unaware. Job actually questions the morality and integrity of God:

> I will say unto God, Do not condemn me; shew me wherefore thou contendest with me. Is it good unto thee that thou shouldest oppress, that thou shouldest despise the work of thine hands, and shine upon the counsel of the wicked? (Job 10:2, 3)

However, when God reproves him at the end of the book, Job responds immediately, saying,

> I know that thou canst do every thing, and that no thought can be withholden from thee. Who is he that hideth counsel without knowledge? therefore have I uttered that I understood not; things too wonderful for me, which I knew not. (Job 42:2-3)

In spite of the fact that Job is an upright man with a perfect heart, the Lord still wishes to expose and deal with certain sins in his life of which he is unaware. The way he does this is with illness. It is interesting to note that when he loses his children and all his possessions he remains composed, but when he becomes ill, it is not long before he complains to God.

We may look at men of God, who walk before the Lord with a perfect heart, and wonder why they should have fallen ill. Even in the greatest man of God there may be sinful attitudes that, though undetected by the individual involved, need dealing with, and God often seeks to correct them with sickness. If the man of God realises the sin causing the illness and confesses it, he will be healed.

The desire of God for every child of His is the same. As Job says:

> But he knoweth the way that I take: when he hath tried me, I shall come forth as gold. (Job 23:10)

8

How does healing come?

If you are sick, the one thing you really want to know is how you can be healed.

The Bible makes it plain that when the Lord Jesus suffered and died on the cross for our sins, he not only dealt with the spiritual consequences of our sin but with the physical consequences as well (i.e. illness).

With his stripes we are healed. (Isaiah 53:5)

There is, therefore, absolute provision for healing which has been paid for by the wounds of the Lord Jesus. It is only by His stripes that we can be healed.

If we have some sickness, it means that we have some sin that the Lord wants to deal with. Therefore, in order to be healed from our sickness we need to get right with God in the matter of our particular sin. It will be some specific attitude or area of sin that we have. If there are various illnesses, there will be various sins.

When we are ill, we may be very frightened and start to panic. There is no need to panic. Just relax and seek the Lord and He will lead you.

When we are ill, we may not feel well enough to seek God. Let me assure you, as soon as you truly start to seek Him in prayer, your symptoms will recede and you will have the strength to draw near to Him. Do not be put off by how you feel before you start – let your symptoms drive you to the Lord. However, this can be very difficult. That is why it is also important to get other Christians to pray for us. We can therefore call upon the elders of the church and upon other Christians to pray for us *(see p. 71)*.

> Is any sick among you? let him call for the elders of the church; and let them pray over him, anointing him with oil in the name of the Lord: and the prayer of faith shall save the sick, and the Lord shall raise him up; and if he have committed sins, they shall be forgiven him. Confess your faults one to another, and pray one for another, that ye may be healed. The effectual fervent prayer of a righteous man availeth much. (James 5:14-16)

The information given below applies both when we are praying alone and when we are being prayed for, but the prayer of others will help to bring us to the point where we can get right with God.

Humility

Before seeking the Lord for healing, it is necessary to draw near to Him. You need to come before Him with a humble heart, to acknowledge that He is perfect in all His ways, that He is just, and that if He has allowed you to become ill, He has seen something that needs correcting. Submit yourself to Him, and allow Him to have His perfect way in you. Acknowledge, too, that 'the heart is deceitful above all things, and desperately wicked: who can know it?' (Jeremiah 17:9). Even though we may think we are right with God and want always to be right with Him, we do not know our own hearts. If God has given an illness, we can be sure that He is revealing and dealing with a sin.

Healing

In order to receive healing, you need to take the following steps.

• Open your heart to God

You need to open up your heart fully to the Holy Spirit and allow Him to search it and reveal all your sins, not just the one causing the disease. If we are to have fellowship with God, seeking Him for healing, we can have nothing spoiling our fellowship with Him. Let everything be brought out into the open, out into the light.

> This then is the message which we have heard of him, and declare unto you, that God is light, and in him is no darkness at all. If we say that we have fellowship with him, and walk in darkness, we lie, and do not the truth: but if we walk in the light, as he is in the light, we have fellowship one with another, and the blood of Jesus Christ his Son cleanseth us from all sin. (John 1:5-7)

There is always a temptation to try to hide sins, to cover them up. If we are to be healed, we need to open up our hearts completely to God and allow Him to deal with every sin in our lives as it comes to mind. As we come increasingly into the light of God by confessing any sins that come to mind, we will have clearer vision for seeing the sin that is causing our illness. As the Psalmist says,

> In thy light shall we see light. (Psalm 36:9)

All sins confessed before the Lord are fully cleansed (I John 1:9).

A useful help in opening our hearts to God and searching them is the extract from Finney's teaching on revival, found in Appendix 2 on page 92. We need to come to the place where all known sin is confessed.

As you seek to draw near to God, you need to remove all worldly influences from your life. Avoid watching television, listening to the radio, reading the newspaper and secular books. This will help you to hear God's voice.

You will also find that fasting is of immense value (*see* Appendix 3: Fasting, *page 102*).

- **Know what the sin is which has caused your sickness**

There is guidance in the latter part of this book about which sins cause which sicknesses. However, although this book may point you in the right direction, your eyes need to be opened to your own sin and situation by the Holy Spirit, so the most important thing is to spend time seeking the Lord in prayer.

It may be helpful to talk to a trusted friend or family member. It is often much easier for others to see our faults than for us. It is likely that the sin which is causing our sickness will be fairly obvious to everyone apart from us.

• Confess it before the Lord

Once you have discovered what the sin is, you need really to acknowledge that it is wrong, and that it is serious, something that has displeased God. Then all you need to do is confess it before the Lord and believe that the blood of Jesus cleanses you from the sin, and you are forgiven. You can then simply ask the Lord to heal you and He will.

Avoid the temptation to play down the sin, to excuse it, to make yourself believe that you don't really commit it. There is no need, since entire provision has been made for its cleansing by the Lord Jesus.

> If we say that we have no sin, we deceive ourselves, and the truth is not in us. If we confess our sins, he is faithful and just to forgive us our sins, and to cleanse us from all unrighteousness. (I John 1:8, 9)

If the sin has truly been confessed, forsaken and cleansed, the sickness will go.

Note also that you cannot remove a sin by trying to stop committing it. Sin is only cleansed by confessing it to God – by admitting that you are guilty of it and trusting Him to forgive you. He then gives you power to stop committing it.

Perseverance

In many cases, the process of seeking the Lord and getting right with Him will take time. Don't be discouraged, but keep seeking Him until you have met with Him and He has revealed your problem and healed you. If this takes days, don't give up.

The willingness of Christ

As Christians, we usually believe that Christ is able to heal us. We believe that He created the heavens and the earth, that he can do anything. We often doubt, however, that He is willing to heal us.

Let me assure you that **Jesus is always willing to heal us**. There may be some issue that is temporarily blocking the healing, but the Lord is still so willing that we should be healed. Inasmuch as He has already paid the price for our healing with His sufferings on the cross, He desires that we should come into the benefit of that provision.

When the leper, in Matthew 8, came to Jesus, he understood that Jesus was able to heal him. The only doubt in his mind was as to whether He was willing. He said to Jesus:

> Lord, if thou wilt, thou canst make me clean. (Matthew 8:2)

Jesus replies:

> I will; be thou clean. (Matthew 8:3)

And to us, in our moment of need, the Lord Jesus says just the same: 'I am willing'.

God is so full of goodness, He wants to bless us and meet our every need. The Lord Jesus is described as being full of grace and truth. *Truth* says, 'I need to deal with your sin issue before you can be healed'. *Grace* says, 'But I am nonetheless so willing to heal you once you repent'.

Later in the same chapter, we find that everyone that came to Jesus for healing was healed.

> When evening came, they brought to him many possessed with demons. He cast out the spirits with a word, and healed all who were sick. (Matthew 8:16)

The Lord was willing in every case.

In seeking our healing we need to believe not only that He can heal us but that He is willing to as well.

9

The role of Elders

In James 5, there is clear instruction that elders have a role to play in healing.

> Is any sick among you? let him call for the elders of the church; and let them pray over him, anointing him with oil in the name of the Lord: and the prayer of faith shall save the sick, and the Lord shall raise him up; and if he have committed sins, they shall be forgiven him. (James 5:14-16)

It may very properly be asked how this works in practice within the context of this doctrine of healing in which sin and sickness are seen to be connected.

First of all it must be noted that the statement 'the prayer of faith shall save the sick, and the Lord shall raise him up' is unequivocal. There is no doubt that a sick individual should be healed when prayed for. It is not the Lord's will that they should remain sick.

However, there appear to be two conditional factors. The first is that the prayer should be in faith. This is a very simple matter and simply means that when prayer is made that the one praying should meet with God. The woman with the issue of blood pressed through the crowd and touched just the hem of the Lord's garment and yet was healed. The person praying needs only to touch heaven in the smallest way.

Loud enthusiastic prayer is not necessary. Choice of words

does not matter. Quoting scripture is not necessary. All that matters is that the one praying meets with God as they do so.

Some people are known to pray in tongues over the sick. This is unnecessary and inappropriate. It comes from the mistaken belief that because the gift of tongues is a supernatural gift, that there is a supernatural power in it. There is not. Praying in an unknown tongue is for the individual's personal edification (I Corinthians 14:4) or is to be used in conjunction with interpretation as a means of God's speaking to the church. It should not be used when praying for the sick.[18]

Secondly, the sin must be dealt with. As the person is being prayed for, the Holy Spirit will be working in him, pressing him to turn from his sin (he may or may not be sensitive to this). If he is open to the Holy Spirit, he may at this point get direct revelation about the issue that needs dealing with and can repent. As he repents he will receive his healing. In many cases, the sin issue may be dealt with by the Holy Spirit in the person's heart, without their fully realising it with the mind. The Holy Spirit simply does a work and the person is healed and spiritually restored. Thus people may be healed without any verbal or mental reference to sin. However, a spiritual change has occured. It will be real and lasting, but the fact that the sin has been forgiven and dealt with has not registered in the mind. The person will simply feel refreshed and spiritually liberated.

As the elder praying meets with God, he should have a sense either that the person will be healed, or that the person's sin has not been dealt with and is blocking the healing. In the latter case, the elder should receive revelation as to the nature of the sin, in order to mention it to the sufferer that they might confess it, be forgiven and healed. If the one that is ill does not receive the revelation for himself, the onus is always on the elders.

And if he have committed sins, they shall be forgiven him. (James 5:16)[19]

---

[18] Of course, when praying for the sick, someone may receive a *message* in an unknown tongue, which should then be interpreted. This may be used by God to reveal to the person the nature of their sin.

[19] For a discussion of the word 'if' in this verse, please see page 24 and footnote 5, page 25.

Lance Lambert tells a useful story in this regard:

> I remember years ago being struck by a story about that great Danish servant of the Lord, Pastor Fjord Christensen. A group of people were called out into the country to pray for a woman who had not been able to walk for a number of years because she was crippled with arthritis. But she was a believer and so was her husband. As they prayed and prayed, a younger man prayed with much zeal and much devotion, but he did not get far. The older man, Fjord Christensen, just said 'Amen' at different points and kept very quiet. He was looking in his Bible. Suddenly, he stopped the prayer and said to the lady, 'Could you tell me, are you short-tempered?'
>
> She was startled and said, 'Oh, no!'
>
> So they continued to pray. Then a little later, he stopped again and said, 'Excuse me asking, but are you quite sure that you are not irritable?'
>
> 'Oh no, never,' she said. 'I never get irritated.'
>
> So they went on praying. Suddenly, he said, 'Are you absolutely certain that you are not short-tempered?'
>
> And when she was about to say 'no', her husband burst in with tears in his eyes and said, 'Oh, but you are! You are! It is the worst thing about you.'
>
> 'Ah,' said Fjord Christensen, 'I thought so.' The woman burst into tears and she confessed to the Lord how short-tempered she was with her husband and everything else. When it was all out of her and she had really repented, Fjord Christensen said, 'Now we can ask the Lord to heal you.' And he read her Proverbs 14:30 which in Danish is translated 'A sound heart is the life of the flesh: but short-temperedness is the rottenness of the bones.'
>
> While they had been praying, this verse had come to Fjord Christensen, and that is why he persisted in his questions until the truth was revealed. When they laid hands on that woman, she stood up and was able to see the men out. She lived a normal life until her death, and never had arthritis again.[20]

This is the normal way it should be when praying for the sick.

---

[20] *Watch and Pray,* Lance Lambert, (Kingsway Publications, 1995), pp.98-99

10

The time of Jacob's trouble

A useful story from scripture to help us understand why God uses physical suffering to correct his children is that of God wrestling with Jacob.

Jacob, throughout his life had been a twister. Everything that he had wanted in life he had acquired by his own cunning. Though the things that he had wanted were worthy, his means had always been wrong.

When in his youth he has a desire for his brother's birthright, he corners Esau at a weak moment and Esau sells it to him for a bowl of lentil pottage.

When Jacob desires his brother's blessing as the first-born, he acquires it by dressing up as Esau and pretending to his blind father that he is his brother.

When Laban offers Jacob wages for looking after his cattle, Jacob asks for all the spotted and speckled cattle. Laban agrees, but then promptly removes all of them and sends them three days' journey away. Jacob, in return, so contrives things after that that all the healthy cattle have spotted and speckled offspring and the weak cattle give birth to plain. He thus manages to gain a great herd of healthy cattle.

However, there comes a time in Jacob's life when he is pushed to his limit. He has just made his peace with Laban and he is on his way to visit his father Isaac in Padanaram. He wants to make peace with Esau, so on the way he sends a message to him asking for grace. His messengers return to say that Esau is on his way with four hundred men.

Jacob is terrified. He has taken Esau's birthright and blessing, and no contact has been made with him since. Now Esau is on his way with four hundred men, and Jacob is surrounded by his family and livestock. He panics.

He takes immediate action by dividing up his family and possessions into two groups so that if he loses one half, he still has the other. He then prays a frantic prayer of unbelief.

> Deliver me, I pray thee, from the hand of my brother, from the hand of Esau: for I fear him, lest he will come and smite me, and the mother with the children. And thou saidst, I will surely do thee good, and make thy seed as the sand of the sea, which cannot be numbered for multitude. (Genesis 32:11, 12)

He then sends a huge gift of livestock on ahead to his brother to pacify him, and then settles down amongst his people for the night. Clearly unable to sleep, he rises in the night and sends his family over the brook into a safer place. He is evidently terrified.

It is when he is in this state of fear and confusion that the Lord enters powerfully into his life once more:

> And Jacob was left alone; and there wrestled a man with him until the breaking of the day. (Genesis 32:24)

Many people claim that this passage is about Jacob wrestling with God, but the verse makes it clear that in the middle of Jacob's great day of trouble, God comes to wrestle with *him*.

God has been patient with Jacob over many years as Jacob has sought to get things though his own means. Instead of trusting God, he has always looked for a clever method of his own; he has always used his own resources. Now he has finally come to the place where trusting himself is nearly sending him mad. So God says, as it were, 'Enough is enough: it's time we dealt with this'. So He comes and wrestles with him.

Still reluctant to let God have his own way, Jacob resists. Then God strikes his body.

> And when he saw that he prevailed not against him, he touched the hollow of his thigh; and the hollow of Jacob's thigh was out of joint, as he wrestled with him. (Genesis 32:25)

The thigh joint is the strongest part of a man's body, so in striking him there, God is fully incapacitating him. However, even though his body has been struck by God, Jacob is determined to carry on living in his own strength. He says:

> Let me go, for the day breaketh.

And God replies:

> I will not let thee go, except thou bless me.

(Most commentators put the above statements into the mouths of the opposite people, so that God says, 'Let me go' and Jacob replies, 'I will not'. However, the Hebrew gives no indication as to who makes which statement, and the context and sense of the passage all favour the rendering I have given.)

As the day is approaching, Jacob is afraid of what is going to happen, and he wants to be up and ready to try and work something out. It is so often the case that we struggle against God, even when he has brought us down to a place of desperation and weakness. But what does God mean when he asks Jacob to bless Him?

It really means to acknowledge who God is. The word for *bless* literally means *to kneel* – in other words, to 'give unto the LORD the glory due unto his name' (Psalm 29:2). Jacob has been in such a panic that he will not acknowledge that God is in control, that He loves him, that he will look after him. He continually tries to do everything in his own strength, not trusting that God will take care of him. So God says in effect, 'This has gone on long enough. I will not let you go unless you acknowledge who I am and start to trust me.'

Then, just as He has struck the strongest part of his body, God now puts His finger on the pivotal part of Jacob's character. He asks 'What is thy name?'

And Jacob replies, 'Jacob.'

In asking Jacob his name, God is really asking Jacob to admit who he is, what he is really like. And his name, meaning 'Supplanter' or 'Twister' says it all.

This was all that God was looking for: an honest admission from Jacob that he has been trying to get everything by twisting, rather than trusting God. Jacob has finally come through. He has overcome. He has got to the place God wanted him to. He has prevailed.

> And he said, Thy name shall be called no more Jacob, but Israel: for as a prince hast thou power with God and with men, and hast prevailed. (Genesis 32:28)

In response to this, Jacob asks the Lord who He is.

> And Jacob asked him, and said, Tell me, I pray thee, thy name. And he said, Wherefore is it that thou dost ask after my name? And he blessed him there. (Genesis 32:29)

In blessing him, God was saying to Jacob, 'This is who I am: I am all that you need', and in so doing, revealed himself to be God, the all-sufficient one.

This is the way the Lord works in all believers

When we become ill, it is for us the time of Jacob's trouble, the time when God wants finally to deal with something that has been making us spiritually lame for years. It will generally be the most difficult part of our character to deal with. As with Jacob, all we need to do is submit to the Lord and acknowledge who we really are, that is to say, confess the sin of our hearts, and the Lord will forgive us our sin and heal us of our illness.

There is a wider application to this as well. When God wants to deal with His church, when Christians have become lax over sin, God will finally say 'Enough is enough. It is time for you to be revived', and He will apply this principle to the whole church. Christians will fall ill in great number as God seeks to bring them back to himself.

In Jeremiah 30, it speaks of the 'time of Jacob's trouble' as it applied to Israel and Judah. It describes men clutching their loins like women in labour, out of utter terror at what is happening. Such was Jacob's fear when Esau was approaching, and such was the fear of Israel and Judah as they went into captivity. God describes the captivity of Israel and Judah as the time of Jacob's trouble since it was the time when He was finally going to deal with their sin.

Yet, throughout, God reiterates that, though there is the chastening, He is with them, and loves them and is doing it for a purpose:

> For I am with thee, saith the LORD, to save thee: though I make a full end of all nations whither I have scattered thee, yet I will not make a full end of thee: but I will correct thee in measure, and will not leave thee altogether unpunished. (Jeremiah 30:11)

Finally, we find the subject returns to that of healing:

> For thus saith the LORD, Thy bruise is incurable, and thy wound is grievous. There is none to plead thy cause, that thou mayest be bound up: thou hast no healing medicines. All thy lovers have forgotten thee; they seek thee not; for I have wounded thee with the wound of an enemy, with the chastisement of a cruel one, for the multitude of thine iniquity; because thy sins were increased. Why criest thou for thine affliction? thy sorrow is incurable for the multitude of thine iniquity: because thy sins were increased, I have done these things unto thee. (Jeremiah 30:12-15)

Here again, we see several themes that have come out again and again: the wound is inflicted by the Lord; it is given because of sin; it appears to be incurable.

Yet in the midst of their affliction, God says:

> For I will restore health unto thee, and I will heal thee of thy wounds, saith the LORD. (Jeremiah 30:17)

Though the wound is incurable to man, 'by His stripes we are healed.'

11

Satan and demons – their role in sickness

As we consider the subject of physical illness, we may ask the question, who makes the person ill – is it God or Satan? The answer to this is found in the book of Job. When Job is smitten, two things are clear: Satan is the one who actually strikes him with illness, but God allows it in order to deal with an issue of sin in his life.

> Satan answered the LORD, and said, Skin for skin, yea, all that a man hath will he give for his life. But put forth thine hand now, and touch his bone and his flesh, and he will curse thee to thy face. And the LORD said unto Satan, Behold, he is in thine hand; but save his life. So went Satan forth from the presence of the LORD, and smote Job with sore boils from the sole of his foot unto his crown. (Job 2:4-7)

Satan previously complains that God has put a hedge of protection around Job which has stopped Satan attacking him.

> Hast not thou made an hedge about him, and about his house, and about all that he hath on every side? thou hast blessed the work of his hands, and his substance is increased in the land. (Job 1:10)

It is obvious then that, in order for Satan to gain access, the hedge must be removed. This means that, when someone falls ill, God has ordained that it should happen, but it is Satan that acts as the agent. It is therefore correct to say that God has given the illness, because it is He who has allowed it, but that Satan is the agent who has actually done it.

Therefore, when a person sins, God removes the hedge of protection and the person can be made physically ill by Satan and his messengers (demons). These demons have access to smite with disease that very part of the body that symbolizes the area of sin, and no other.

Demons and temptation

To understand more fully the role of Satan and demons in illness, it needs to be realized that not only do they make a person ill when he sins, but that they are the ones who tempt the person to sin in the first place.

> Let no man say when he is tempted, I am tempted of God: for God cannot be tempted with evil, neither tempteth he any man. (James 1:13)

Satan always wants to destroy, so he tempts people to sin, and once they have succumbed to temptation, he condemns them and smites them with illness. And yet God, in His sovereignty allows all of this for His own purposes and for our good. As we learn to overcome temptation, we become stronger and more mature spiritually, and we learn something of what it means to reign with Christ.

What about demons in people?

The subject of demons seems to arouse two extremes of opinion. Generally people either dismiss any notion that they can powerfully affect a person's life, or they suggest that demons can operate in a person's life completely irrespective of that person's lifestyle and sin. I believe both stances are incorrect.

The existence of demons and their effect upon certain people is clear from Scripture. Indeed, when the Lord Jesus went about ministering, casting out demons was done alongside healing.

> And he healed many that were sick of divers diseases, and cast out many devils. (Mark 1:34)

Whilst we are fully aware of physical sickness today, the idea of demonic activity is often overlooked. And yet dealing with it was a key part of Christ's commission to His disciples:

> Heal the sick, cleanse the lepers, raise the dead, cast out devils: freely ye have received, freely give. (Matthew 10:8)

Moreover, the Lord does not limit this to the disciples. He says:

> And these signs shall follow them that believe; in my name shall they cast out devils. (Mark 16:17)

Since there were demons in the Lord's day and in the time of the Apostles, we must accept that they are still present and active today.

How demons operate

Demons begin by attacking an individual with temptation. Once the person succumbs, they have a foothold in that person's life, and three things happen: 1) they condemn the person, discouraging him and making him think there is no hope for him. This, they intend, will lead the person to give up spiritually, and so fall completely into sin. 2) The person loses the victory in this one area of sin and will not be able to stop himself repeating it. Demons are able to cause the person to commit the sin over and over again, and he has no power to resist. 3) The Lord may permit them to strike the person's body.

Although demons have power to affect someone after he has sinned, the Christian can regain the victory simply by confessing the sin and getting right with God.

> If we confess our sins, he is faithful and just to forgive us our sins, and to cleanse us from all unrighteousness. (I John 1:9)

If we confess our sins, God cleanses us from them, and the demon has lost the ability to touch us, either to condemn us, to make us sin, or to smite us physically.

Demon influence and control over people

Therefore, the subject of demon influence is really very simple. It is a matter of whom we allow to control our lives. Paul says,

> To whom ye yield yourselves servants to obey, his servants ye are to whom ye obey; whether of sin unto death, or of obedience unto righteousness. (Romans 6:16)

When we sin, it means we have succumbed to temptation and have therefore chosen to submit to the devil rather than to submit to God. We are choosing to serve sin, and therefore to serve the purposes of the devil. We have given him control over an area of our lives and we cannot break free from this control while the sin remains. However, the devil can only control us in that area that we have yielded to him (for example, in the area of a bad temper). He can keep us committing the same sin but not other sins.

Now, the more we yield to the devil, the more control he has over our lives. There are certain things, therefore, that give demons full access to control a person and dominate his life. If a person willingly enters into communion with darkness, he is putting his whole life into the hands of demons. They can then dominate him and run his life. This is often termed demon possession.

There are three particular ways in which demons are enabled to possess a person:

• Through wilful active communion with evil spirits, such as through occultism, spiritism, mind-reading, astrology and horoscopes, fortune telling, freemasonry and worship of false gods.

• Through mind-altering drugs. A person who takes such drugs is actively seeking an experience of something unknown to themselves, which in reality is an experience of demonic activity.

• Through fornication. When a person joins their body

to another, he becomes one flesh with that person: they are having spiritual communion (I Corinthians 6:16). The only time God sanctions sexual activity is within the context of a marriage between a man and a woman. Other sexual practice, such as adultery or prostitution, opens a person up to demon possession. (Note also that marrying a divorced person or remarrying after divorce can count as adultery – see Luke 16:18).

Now the primary way of breaking free from demon control remains the same with demon possession. If the person confesses to God their sin, the devil immediately loses control over that person's life.

In some cases, however, the person is so controlled by demons that they cannot break free on their own. In such cases, outside help will be necessary. A Christian can therefore command the demon to leave the person in the name of Jesus. After this has happened, the person should come to God for cleansing and infilling with the Holy Spirit.

What are the signs of demon control?

LEVEL 1 – DEMON INFLUENCE

At a basic level, every time a person has a sin problem in a particular area, it means that they have lost the victory in that area and demons are able to keep the person sinning. This is an everyday occurrence, a feature of the lives of all Christian believers. Once the sin is identified, it can be confessed and the demon loses its foothold.

LEVEL 2 – DEMON POSSESSION

Demon possession may be evident in two ways. Firstly, when someone's life is marked by wickedness, we can observe that they are fully controlled by demons. There may be nothing obviously bizarre in their behaviour, but they are being used by Satan. They will typically be seen actively to do evil, such as breaking up relationships, wilfully hindering Christian work, or causing damage in other ways. This active evil differs from the normal sinfulness that every human displays. A scriptural example of this is Elymas the sorcerer (Acts 13:6-11).

Secondly, however, there may be extreme manifestations, and these are the people that need outside help. Examples of these are given in the Bible and there appear to be three main manifestations.

• Extreme physical behaviour (this obviously differs from illnesses such as epilepsy).

And as he was yet a coming, the devil threw him down, and tare him. And Jesus rebuked the unclean spirit, and healed the child, and delivered him again to his father. (Luke 9:42)

• Demons speaking through the person.

And it came to pass, as we went to prayer, a certain damsel possessed with a spirit of divination met us, which brought her masters much gain by soothsaying: the same followed Paul and us, and cried, saying, These men are the servants of the most high God, which shew unto us the way of salvation. (Acts 16:16-17)

• Indwelling demons can also be manifest by physical illness and disability.

And he was casting out a devil, and it was dumb. And it came to pass, when the devil was gone out, the dumb spake; and the people wondered. (Luke 11:14)

Mental illness
In all cases, mental illness is an indication of demon activity, though it may come from level 1 (demon influence) or level 2 (demon possession).

How to deal with demons
A. DEMON OPPRESSION
When demons are merely oppressing a person, tempting him to sin, they can be resisted. They may bring difficulties your way, and cause hardship, but they have no power over you; they cannot influence or control you.

Resist the devil, and he will flee from you. (James 4:7)

It may be helpful in such cases to speak out against the devil as the Lord did, quoting Scripture and telling him to go. (Luke 4:1-7)

B. DEMON INFLUENCE AND DEMON POSSESSION

When demons have gained some level of control over a person, they need to be dealt with. In all cases, demons can only control or influence a person when there is sin in a person's life. If you deal with the sin, by confession to God and receiving the cleansing of the blood, you also deal with the demon. This is nearly always the way to deal with a demon.

The only time for other measures is when a person is so controlled that they are not in a position to confess their sin and get right with God. In such cases, a Christian, acting under the authority of the Lord Jesus, is able to cast them out by speaking to them.

When the Lord Jesus was on earth, He cast demons out of people again and again and he gave authority to both his disciples and to all subsequent believers to cast them out (Mark 16:17). Therefore any Christian should be able to cast out demons.

Important conditions

There are two main conditions which may determine whether a Christian is in a position to cast out a demon. **First, he must be at that moment under the authority of the Lord Jesus.** He can only have authority over demons if he is himself under authority, since authority is delegated (see Luke 7:8). If, for example, there is unconfessed sin in his life, he will have no authority and therefore no power over demons. For this reason, it may be necessary to be regularly in prayer and fasting in order to be in a sufficient place of spiritual rightness with God.

And when he was come into the house, his disciples asked him privately, Why could not we cast him out? And he said unto them, This kind can come forth by nothing, but by prayer and fasting. (Mark 9:28:29)

Secondly, he must cast them out in the name of Jesus. The Christian does not have his own authority to cast out demons – it is only in the name of Jesus that he acts and speaks.

An example from Scripture

A model example of how to cast out a demon is found in Acts 16. Paul is being followed by a girl possessed by an evil spirit, who cries out,

> These men are the servants of the most high God, which shew unto us the way of salvation. (Acts 16:17)

In response, Paul casts the demon out.

> Paul, being grieved, turned and said to the spirit, I command thee in the name of Jesus Christ to come out of her. And he came out the same hour. (Acts 16:18)

From this we can learn several things. First, that Paul spoke directly to the evil spirit. He did not speak to the girl, but to the evil spirit within the girl. Secondly, he did not pray that the spirit should go, but directly commanded the spirit itself. Thirdly, he commands the spirit 'in the name of Jesus Christ'.

Other facts we learn from Scripture are that demons may argue, they will be reluctant to come out, and that there may be numerous demons inside a person. We discover this from Luke 8.

> And when he went forth to land, there met him out of the city a certain man, which had devils long time, and ware no clothes, neither abode in any house, but in the tombs. When he saw Jesus, he cried out, and fell down before him, and with a loud voice said, What have I to do with thee, Jesus, thou Son of God most high? I beseech thee, torment me not. (For he had commanded the unclean spirit to come out of the man. For oftentimes it had caught him: and he was kept bound with chains and in fetters; and he brake the bands, and was driven of the devil into the wilderness.) And Jesus asked him, saying, What is thy name? And he said, Legion: because many devils

were entered into him. And they besought him that he would
not command them to go out into the deep. And there was
there an herd of many swine feeding on the mountain: and they
besought him that he would suffer them to enter into them. And
he suffered them. Then went the devils out of the man, and
entered into the swine: and the herd ran violently down a steep
place into the lake, and were choked. (Luke 8:27-33)

We observe that, although the demons were numerous and
although they argued, ultimately they had to submit to the
authority of Christ.

Appendix 1

What about doctors?

Extract from *The Gifts of the Spirit,* by Harold Horton: Chapter 12 – The Gifts of Healing

Harold Horton *was one of the great Pentecostal leaders and teachers of the first half of the twentieth century. His book,* The Gifts of the Spirit, *led the way in reteaching Pentecostal truths to the church.*

Gifts of Healings are commonly confused with a high degree of medical or surgical or manipulative or scientific ability. These are all of the natural man. They do not occur in the Scriptures at all, except as they are superseded in Christ. Healings through these Gifts are wrought by the power of Christ through the Spirit, by ignorant believers. True, Luke the beloved physician was among the Lord's disciples. So was John the beloved fisherman. As the one became a spiritual fisher and supernatural healer, so the other became a supernatural healer and spiritual fisher. It is entirely dishonest to suggest as some writers do that Paul took Luke with him on his journeys as a safeguard, in case his miraculous Gifts failed! Those who know God's miraculous ways in the Scriptures look upon such a statement as an impossible travesty of the truth. For all God's Miracle-Gifts work only according to faith. Means, such as Luke's supposititious medicine chest, are the very opposite of faith. Unbelief, in short.

The Gifts of the Spirit do not work with means but without them. The sin in Abraham that delayed the birth of Isaac until it was put away was the 'means' he provided as a resort in case the miracle of the promise failed to work. While Hagar was behind the door, so to speak, as an aid to God in the fulfilment of His promise that promise could not possibly be fulfilled. The miracle eventually transpired, not through expedients or partial means, but through faith alone. When Luke the physician followed Jesus he no longer used medicines and media; he healed like the other disciples (if he healed at all) by the laying on of hands and anointing with oil. When Paul and Luke, and others, arrived at the island of Melita and found people desperately sick, it was not Luke the physician with his medicine chest who healed them, but Paul the tent-maker by the laying on of hands and the working of these mighty gifts.[21]

While we hope we should be among the last to speak disparagingly of hospitals, or of doctors and nurses who give so unsparingly of their time and efforts for the alleviation of human suffering, yet we must most emphatically state that modern medicine is not the legitimate fulfilment of Jesus' command to 'heal the sick'. Rather is it the negation, the neglect, if not the positive denial of it. And this is equally true of genuinely born-again 'Christian doctors'. The only 'Christian physicians' acknowledged in the Scriptures are those ordinary believers who heal miraculously through these Gifts, or equally miraculously through the laying on of hands or anointing with oil. The supposition that the Lord Jesus heals today through Harley Street is no more Scriptural than the claim that He saves through Oxford. Medicine and surgery is the world's way. God's way, the only way revealed in the Word, is healing by supernatural divine power. These two ways are entirely opposed. True, many real Christians resort to the way of the unbeliever, but that does not alter the fact that it is the way of the unbeliever. Divine healing is the only healing authorised by the Scriptures. Medical healing is not, as some people declare, 'God's second best'. It is entirely of the educated world. God has no second best.

In an ultimate sense, of course, all healing is of God. But then in this ultimate sense all sickness is likewise of God, and all everything else, except sin. 'I kill, and I make alive; I wound, and I heal' is Jehovah's declaration (Deut. 32:39). 'In faithfulness hast thou afflicted me' admits the Psalmist.

If medical practice were really the continuation of Christ's

---

[21] There is no reason to suppose that Luke continued to practise medicine after he began serving the Lord. Matthew the publican and Simon the leper both retain their epithets after the latter cease to apply (see Matt. 10:3 and 26:6).

beneficent work, as in many quarters it is claimed to be, the work would be done freely, as the preaching of the gospel ought still to be, as both actually were in the Lord Jesus' day and in the day of the early Christians. True the labourer (workman) is worthy of his hire (meat). But that 'hire' in the Scripture never means more than bread for the hour. Then how can doctors claim that they are doing the Lord's work when they neither serve Him nor believe in Him in many cases, and when they unblushingly call in the aid of the Christ-rejecting world in support of their work and efforts? Can the holy Lord really receive the gains of ungodly 'sweepstakes' and stage-celebrity auctions and music hall iniquities? And how can a man who knows how such money is raised call himself a Christian doctor while he has part in such ungodly methods, and fellowship with such unscrupulous men on equal terms without protest? Has the Lord really given over His beloved sick to the world, and His precious Gifts of Healing to the ungodly who reject His grace daily and even blaspheme His holy Name?

Believers will recall two attractive pictures, illustrating Christ the Saviour and Christ the Healer respectively. Do they ever notice the inconsistency in comparison? The Saviour picture shows a number of lovely children clambering happily around the seated Christ. Beautiful. The other, however, shows a number of sick children with one obviously ready to die in the foreground. But this time instead of the Christ there is a young doctor in white overalls with his ugly instruments and phials exposed at his feet, and the Lord Jesus a shadowy figure in the background! Is not this an exact representation of the position of Christ in the healing of men today? But to make these two pictures agree ought not the Christ, not the doctor, to be the prominent figure as the Healer, with the sick children being healed as of old by His divine touch alone, even as the lost are saved by His divine hand alone? Or the other way about, ought not the happy children in the Saviour picture to be clambering round a nun or a priest with Christ a shadowy figure in the background — as He actually is today, in many quarters, with regard both to salvation and healing?

No thinking person can really believe that poisonous drugs and cruel scalpels have anything to do with divine healing. To put it quite reasonably, with no shadow of intended offence, surely medicine at its best is merely a development of the world's ever-changing and ever-futile attempts to wipe out disease. As this generation laughs at the methods of the last, surely a wise man can see that the next generation will laugh (if the Lord tarry) at the methods of today. Is it not obvious that the Lord God has His hand on the world? And is it not possible that He Himself wonders at human attempts to rid the world of disease — in order that ungodly men might be at ease in ignoring Him and mocking at His blessed Son and His merciful salvation? And is the world really more healthy today after all men's efforts than it was when our grandparents lived? Is it not just that as one disease begins to relax its mortifying hold another more terrible most relentlessly adjusts its grasp?

The Lord still has compassion on the sick. He still has a way of deliverance from the power of the enemy. It is still the way revealed in His Word. The sick do well to seek it out and bring their diseases to Him as the distressed their maladies of old. It is the safe way; a painless way; a free way and a holy way. Because it is His way.

Appendix 2

Breaking up the fallow ground
Extract from *Lectures on Revival* by Charles Finney.

Note: Finney frequently refers to 'religion' and 'professors'. By 'religion' he always means Christianity, by 'professors', he means Christians, or those who profess to be Christians.

> Break up your fallow ground: for it is time to seek the Lord, till He come and rain righteousness upon you. (Hosea 10:12)

The Jews were a nation of farmers, and it is therefore a common thing in the Scriptures to refer for illustrations to their occupation, and to the scenes with which farmers and shepherds are familiar. The prophet Hosea addresses them as a nation of backsliders; he reproves them for their idolatry, and threatens them with the judgments of God.

A revival consists of two parts: as it respects the Church, and as it respects the ungodly. I shall speak on this occasion of a revival in the Church. Fallow ground is ground which has once been tilled, but which now lies waste, and needs to be broken up and mellowed, before it is suited to receive grain.

If you mean to break up the fallow ground of your hearts, you must begin by looking at your hearts: examine and note the state of your minds, and see where you are. Many never seem to think about this. They pay no attention to their own hearts, and never know whether they are doing well in religion or not; whether they are gaining ground or going back; whether they are fruitful, or lying waste. Now you must draw off your attention from other things, and look into this. Make a business of it. Do not be in a hurry. Examine thoroughly the state of your hearts, and see where you are: whether you are walking with God every day, or with the devil.

Self-examination consists in looking at your lives, in considering your actions, in calling up the past, and learning its true character. Look back over your past history. Take up your individual sins one by one, and look at them. I do not mean that you should just cast a glance at your past life, and see that it has been full of sins, and then go to God and make a sort of general confession, and ask for pardon. That is not the way. You must take them up one by one. It will be a good thing to take a pen and paper, as you go over them and write them down as they occur to you.

Go over them as carefully as a merchant goes over his books; and as often as a sin comes before your memory, add it to the list. General confessions of sin will never do. Your sins were committed one by one; and as far as you can come at them, they ought to be reviewed and repented of one by one. Now begin, and take up first what are commonly, but improperly, called Sins of Omission.

1. *Ingratitude.* Take this sin, for instance, and write down under that head all the instances you can remember wherein you have

received favours from God for which you have never exercised gratitude. How many cases can you remember? Some remarkable providence, some wonderful turn of events, that saved you from ruin. Set down the instances of God's goodness to you when you were in sin, before your conversion, for which you have never been half thankful enough; and the numerous mercies you have received since. How long the catalogue of instances, where your ingratitude has been so black that you are forced to hide your face in confusion! Go on your knees and confess them one by one to God, and ask forgiveness. The very act of confession, by the laws of suggestion, will bring up others to your memory. Put down these! Go over them three or four times in this way, and see what an astonishing number of mercies there are for which you have never thanked God.

2. *Want of love to God.* Think how grieved and alarmed you would be if you discovered any flagging of affection for you in your wife, husband, or children; if you saw another engrossing their hearts, and thoughts, and time. Perhaps in such a case you would well nigh die with a just and virtuous jealousy. Now, God calls Himself a jealous God; and have you not given your heart to other loves and infinitely offended Him?

3. *Neglect of the Bible.* Put down the cases when for perhaps weeks, or longer, God's Word was not a pleasure. Some people, indeed, read over whole chapters in such a way that they could not tell what they had been reading. If so, no wonder that your life is spent at random, and that your religion is such a miserable failure.

4. *Unbelief.* Recall the instances in which you have virtually charged the God of truth with lying, by your unbelief of His express promises and declarations. God has promised to give the Holy Spirit to them that ask Him. Now, have you believed this? Have you expected Him to answer? Have you not virtually said in your hearts, when you prayed for the Holy Spirit: 'I do not believe that I shall receive'? If you have not believed nor expected to receive the blessing which God has expressly promised, you have charged Him with lying.

5. *Neglect of prayer.* Think of the times when you have neglected secret prayer, family prayer, and prayer-meetings; or have prayed in such a way as more grievously to offend God than to have omitted it altogether.

6. *Neglect of the means of grace.* When you have suffered trifling excuses to prevent your attending meetings, have neglected and poured contempt upon the means of salvation, merely from disrelish of spiritual duties.

7. *The manner in which you have performed those duties.* That is, with want of feeling and want of faith, in a worldly frame of mind, so that your words were nothing but a mere chattering of a wretch who did not deserve that God should feel the least care for him. When you have fallen down upon your knees and 'said your prayers' in such an unfeeling and careless manner that if you had been put under oath five minutes after you could not have said for what you had been praying.

8. *Want of love for the souls of your fellow-men.* Look round upon your friends and relatives, and remember how little compassion you have felt for them. You have stood by and seen them going right to hell, and it seems as though you did not care. How many days have there been, in which you have failed to make their condition the subject of a single fervent prayer, or to evince any ardent desire for their salvation?

9. *Want of care for the heathen.* Perhaps you have not cared enough for them to attempt to learn their condition; perhaps not even to take a missionary magazine. Look at this, and see how much you really care for the heathen, and set down honestly the real amount of your feelings for them, and your desire for their salvation. Measure your desire for their salvation. Measure your desire for their salvation by the self-denial you practice, in giving your substance to send them the Gospel. Do you retrench your style of living, and scruple not to subject yourself to any inconvenience to save them? Do you daily pray for them in private? Are you laying by something to put into the treasury of the Lord when you go up to pray? If you are not doing these things, and if your soul is not agonised for the poor benighted heathen, why are you such a hypocrite as to pretend to be a Christian? Why, your profession is an insult to Jesus Christ!

10. *Neglect of family duties.* Think of how you have lived before your family, how you have prayed, what an example you have set before them. What direct efforts do you habitually make for their spiritual good? What duty have you *not* neglected?

11. *Neglect of watchfulness over your own life.* In how many

instances you have hurried over your private duties, and have neither taken yourself to task, nor honestly made up your accounts with God; how often have you entirely neglected to watch your conduct, and, having been off your guard, have sinned before the world, and before the Church, and before God!

12. *Neglect to watch over your brethren.* How often have you broken your covenant that you would watch over them in the Lord? How little do you know or care about the state of their souls? And yet you are under a solemn duty to watch over them. What have you done to make yourself acquainted with them? In how many of them have you interested yourself, to know their spiritual state? Go over the list, and wherever you find there has been a neglect, write it down. How many times have you seen your brethren growing cold in religion, and have not spoken to them about it? You have seen them beginning to neglect one duty after another, and you did not reprove them, in a brotherly way. You have seen them falling into sin, and you let them go on. And yet you pretend to love them. What a hypocrite! Would you see your wife or child going into disgrace, or falling into the fire, and hold your peace? No, you would not. What do you think of yourself, then, to pretend to love Christians (and to love Christ) while you see them going into disgrace, and yet say nothing to them?

13. *Neglect of self-denial.* There are many professors who are willing to do almost anything in religion, that does not require self-denial. But when they are required to do anything that requires them to deny themselves – oh, that is too much! They think they are doing a great deal for God, and doing about as much as He ought in reason to ask if they are only doing what they can do just as well as not; but they are not willing to deny themselves any comfort or convenience whatever for the sake of serving the Lord. They will not willingly suffer reproach for the name of Christ. Nor will they deny themselves the luxuries of life, to save a world from hell. So far are they from remembering that self-denial is a condition of discipleship that they do not know what self-denial is. They never have really denied themselves a riband or a pin for Christ and the Gospel. Oh, how soon such professors will be in hell! Some are giving of their abundance, and are giving much, and are ready to complain that others do not give more; when, in truth, they do not themselves give anything that they need,

anything that they could enjoy if they kept it. They only give of their surplus wealth; and perhaps that poor woman who puts in her mite has exercised more self-denial than they have in giving thousands.

From these we now turn to Sins of Commission.

14. *Worldly mindedness.* What has been the state of your heart in regard to your worldly possessions? Have you looked at them as really yours – as if you had a right to dispose of them as your own, according to your own will? If you have, write that down. If you have loved property, and sought after it for its own sake, or to gratify lust or ambition, or a worldly spirit, or to lay it up for your families, you have sinned, and must repent.

15. *Pride.* Recollect all the instances you can, in which you have detected yourself in the exercise of pride. Vanity is a particular form of pride. How many times have you detected yourself in consulting vanity about your dress and appearance? How many times have you thought more, and taken more pains, and spent more time about decorating your body to go to Church, than you have about preparing your mind for the worship of God? You have gone caring more as to how you appeared outwardly, in the sight of mortal man, than how your soul appeared in the sight of the heart-searching God. You have, in fact, set up yourself to be worshipped by them, rather than prepared to worship God yourself. You sought to divide the worship of God's house, to draw off the attention of God's people to look at your pretty appearance. It is in vain to pretend, now, that you do not care anything about having people look at you. Be honest about it! Would you take all this pain about your looks if every person were blind?

16. *Envy.* Look at the cases in which you were envious of those whom you thought were above you in any respect. Or perhaps you have envied those who have been more talented or more useful than yourself. Have you not so envied some, that you have been pained to hear them praised? It has been more agreeable to you to dwell upon their faults than upon their virtues, upon their failures than upon their successes. Be honest with yourself; and if you have harboured this spirit of hell, repent deeply before God, or He will never forgive you.

17. *Censoriousness.* Instances in which you have had a bitter spirit, and spoken of Christians in a manner devoid of charity

and love; of charity, which requires you always to hope the best the case will admit, and to put the best construction upon any ambiguous conduct.

18. *Slander.* The times you have spoken behind people's backs of the faults, real or supposed, of members of the Church or others, unnecessarily, or without good reason. This is slander. You need not lie to be guilty of slander: to tell the truth with the design to injure is slander.

19. *Levity.* How often have you trifled before God as you would not have dared to trifle in the presence of an earthly sovereign? You have either been an atheist, and forgotten that there was a God, or have had less respect for Him, and His presence, than you would have had for an earthly judge.

20. *Lying.* Understand now what lying is. Any species of designed deception. If the deception be not designed, it is not lying. But if you design to make an impression contrary to the naked truth, you lie. Put down all those cases you can recollect. Do not call them by any soft names. God calls them LIES, and charges you with LYING, and you had better charge yourself correctly. How innumerable are the falsehoods perpetuated every day in business, and in social intercourse, by words, and looks, and actions, designed to make an impression on others, for selfish reasons that are contrary to the truth!

21. *Cheating.* Set down all the cases in which you have dealt with an individual, and done to him that which you would not like to have done to you. That is cheating. God has laid down a rule in the case: 'All things whatsoever ye would that men should do to you, do ye even so to them.' That is the rule. And if you have not done so you are a cheat. Mind, the rule is not that you should do 'what you might reasonably expect them to do to you', for that is a rule which would admit of every degree of wickedness. But it is: 'As ye WOULD they should do to you.'

22. *Hypocrisy.* For instance, in your prayers and confessions to God. Set down the instances in which you have prayed for things you did not really want. And the evidence is, that when you have done praying, you could not tell for what you had prayed. How many times have you confessed sins that you did not mean to break off, and when you had no solemn purpose not to repeat them? Yes, you have confessed sins when you knew you as much

expected to go and repeat them, as you expected to live.

23. *Robbing God.* Think of the instances in which you have misspent your time, squandering the hours which God gave you to serve Him and save souls, in vain amusements or foolish conversation, in reading novels or doing nothing; cases where you have misapplied your talents and powers of mind; where you have squandered money on your lusts, or spent it for things which you did not need, and which did not contribute to your health, comfort, or usefulness. Perhaps some of you have laid out God's money for tobacco. I will not speak of intoxicating drink, for I presume there is no professor of religion here that would drink it; and I hope there is not one that uses that filthy poison, tobacco. Think of a professor of religion using God's money to poison himself with tobacco!

24. *Bad Temper.* Perhaps you have abused your wife, or your children, or your family, or servants, or neighbours. Write it all down.

25. *Hindering others from being useful.* Perhaps you have weakened their influence by insinuations against them. You have not only robbed God of your own talents, but tied the hands of somebody else. What a wicked servant is he who not only loiters himself but hinders the rest! This is done sometimes by taking their time needlessly; sometimes by destroying Christian confidence in them. Thus you have played into the hands of Satan, and not only showed yourself an idle vagabond, but prevented others from working.

If you find you have committed a fault against an individual, and that individual is within your reach, go and confess it immediately, and get that out of the way. If the individual you have injured is too far off for you to go and see him, sit down and write him a letter confessing the injury. If you have defrauded anybody, send the money, the full amount and the interest.

Go thoroughly to work in all this! Go now! Do not put it off; that will only make the matter worse. Confess to God those sins that have been committed against God, and to man, those sins that have been committed against man. Do not think of getting off by going round the stumbling-blocks. Take them up out of the way. In breaking up your fallow ground, you must remove every obstruction. Things may be left that you think little things, and you may wonder why you do not feel as you wish to feel in religion, when the reason is that your proud and carnal mind has covered up something which God required you to confess and remove. Break up all the ground and turn it over. Do not 'balk' it, as the farmers say; do not turn aside for little difficulties; drive the plough right through them, beam deep, and turn the ground up, so that it may all be mellow and soft, and fit to receive the seed and bear fruit an 'hundredfold.'

26. When you have gone over your whole history in this way, thoroughly, if you will then go over the ground the second time, and give your solemn and fixed attention to it, you will find that the things you have put down will suggest other things of which you have been guilty, connected with them or near them. Then go over it a third time, and you will recollect other things connected with these. And you will find in the end that you can remember an amount of history, and particular actions, even in this life, which you did not think you would remember in eternity. Unless you take up your sins in this way, and consider them in detail, one by one, you can form no idea of the amount of them. You should go over the list as thoroughly, and as carefully, and as solemnly, as you would if you were just preparing yourself for the judgment. As you go over the catalogue of your sins, be sure to resolve upon present and *entire* reformation. Wherever you find anything wrong, resolve at once, *in the strength of God, to sin no more in that way.* It will be of no benefit to examine yourself, unless you determine to amend in every particular that which you find wrong in heart, temper, or conduct.

If you find, as you go on with this duty, that your mind is still all dark, cast about you, and you will find there is some reason for the Spirit of God to depart from you. You have not been faithful and thorough. In the progress of such a work you have got to do violence to yourself and bring yourself as a rational being up to this work, with the Bible before you, and try your heart till you *do* feel. You need not expect that God will work a miracle for you to break up your fallow ground. It is to be done by means. Fasten your attention to the subject of your sins. You cannot look at your sins long and thoroughly and see how bad they are, without feeling and feeling deeply.

Experience fully proves the benefit of going over our history in this way. Set yourself to the work now; resolve that you will never stop till you find you can pray. You never will have the Spirit of God dwelling in you till you have unravelled this whole mystery of iniquity, and spread out your sins before God. Let there be this deep work of repentance and full confession, this breaking down before God, and you will have as much of the spirit of prayer as your body can bear up under. The reason why so few Christians know anything about the spirit of prayer is because they never would take the pains to examine themselves properly, and so never knew what it was to have their hearts all broken up in this way.

27. It will do no good to preach to you while your hearts are in this hardened, and waste, and fallow state. The farmer might just as well sow his grain on the rock. It will bring forth no fruit. This is the reason why there are so many fruitless professors in the Church, and why there is so much outside machinery and so little deep-toned feeling. Look at the Sabbath-school, for instance, and see how much machinery there is and how little of the power of Godliness. If you go on in this way the Work of God will continue to harden you, and you will grow worse and worse, just as the rain and snow on an old fallow field make the turf thicker and the clods stronger.

28. Professors of religion should never satisfy themselves, or expect a revival, just by starting out of their slumbers, and blustering about, and talking to sinners. They must get their fallow ground broken up. It is utterly unphilosophical to think of getting engaged in religion in this way. If your fallow ground is broken up, then the way to get more feeling is to go out and see sinners on the road to hell, and talk to them, and guide inquiring souls. Then you will get more feeling. You may get into an excitement without this breaking up; you may show a kind of zeal, but it will not last long, and it will not take hold of sinners, unless your hearts are broken up. The reason is, that you go about mechanically, and have not broken up your fallow ground.

29. And now, finally, will you break up your fallow ground? Will you enter upon the course now pointed out and persevere till you are thoroughly awake? If you fail here, if you do not do this, and get prepared, you can go no farther with me. I have gone

with you as far as it is of any use to go until your fallow ground is broken up.

Now you must make thorough work upon this point, or all I have further to say will do you little good. Nay, it will only harden, and make you worse. If you do not set about this work immediately I shall take it for granted that you do not mean to be revived, that you have forsaken your minister, and mean to let him go up to battle alone. If you do not do this, I charge you with having forsaken Christ, with refusing to repent and do your first works.

Appendix 3

Fasting

Fasting is throughout the Bible a thing that accompanies prayer, repentance and serious seeking after God. It entails going without food (and in some cases water as well) for a prolonged period (at least a day).

In my own experience it has been a thing of immense power in transforming my spiritual life and in freeing me from fleshly attitudes. It adds tremendous power to prayer.

It was a key part of the lives of the Lord Jesus (Matthew 4:2), Moses (Exodus 34:28), David (II Samuel 12) and Paul (II Corinthians 11:27). The point of fasting is that you are casting yourself utterly upon God; you are depriving yourself of physical food so that God becomes your source of sustenance; you are depriving yourself of physical strength so that God becomes your strength. It is a way of dying to self, of crucifying the flesh so that you can walk in the spirit.

The key principles of fasting should be noted:

- It indicates repentance and a serious attitude towards God:

And I set my face unto the Lord God, to seek by prayer and supplications, with fasting, and sackcloth, and ashes: And I prayed unto the LORD my God, and made my confession. (Daniel 9:3-4)

- It enables you to hear the Lord's voice clearly.

As they ministered to the Lord, and fasted, the Holy Ghost said, Separate me Barnabas and Saul for the work whereunto I have called them. (Acts 13:2)

- It should be a normal part of a Christian's lifestyle and should be accompanied by refraining from all the normal pleasures of life:

Defraud ye not one the other, except it be with consent for a time, that ye may give yourselves to fasting and prayer; and come together again, that Satan tempt you not for your incontinency. (I Corinthians 7:5)

- It should be done in secret, but is rewarded by God:

Moreover when ye fast, be not, as the hypocrites, of a sad countenance: for they disfigure their faces, that they may appear unto men to fast. Verily I say unto you, They have their reward. But thou, when thou fastest, anoint thine head, and wash thy face; That thou appear not unto men to fast, but unto thy Father which is in secret: and thy Father, which seeth in secret, shall reward thee openly. (Matthew 6:16-18)

- It can be done in the flesh, for wrong reasons:

Behold, ye fast for strife and debate, and to smite with the fist of wickedness. (Isaiah 58:4)

Practical points

A normal person can fast without it affecting their health for forty days and forty nights. In most circumstances Christians will only need to fast for between one day and a week. Seek guidance from the Lord as to the length of your fast.

The more you fast, the easier it becomes. If you fast for one day the first time, the next time you will be able to increase to three days, then five, then seven.

Decide before you start the length of your fast and determine to stick to that. You may be strongly tempted to stop after a short time.

No form of nutrition should be consumed, so drink only water. Drink plenty of water.

The point of the fast is to deprive yourself of normal pleasures so that you can give yourself wholly to God. You should therefore refrain from thinking about food, especially the food you may eat when finishing the fast.

Since during the fast you are replacing physical food with spiritual food (the Lord Jesus Himself) it will help you to get through the fast to spend as much time in fellowship with the Lord as possible. Don't think about the fact that you are fasting – switch off about it and relax, and you will find it is easy.

Fasting weakens the body. If your occupation involves hard physical labour, it may be wise to fast when you have time off from work.

Beware – fasting usually causes bad breath during the fast.

Appendix 4

Further Questions from Scripture

In Matthew 8, it quotes Isaiah 53:4 that the Lord Jesus 'Himself took our infirmities, and bare our sicknesses.' This is clearly referring to the Lord's earthly healing ministry. Doesn't this mean that healing is not provided to every believer through the work of the cross?

The passage in Matthew 8 does indeed state that the Lord's earthly healing ministry was the fulfilment of the prophecy in Isaiah:

> When the even was come, they brought unto him many that were possessed with devils: and he cast out the spirits with his word, and healed all that were sick: that it might be fulfilled which was spoken by Esaias the prophet, saying, Himself took our infirmities, and bare our sicknesses. (Matthew 8:16-17)

Yet we know that all the blessings that came to believers before

Christ had died were paid for by His death on the cross. Every believer under the old covenant received forgiveness of sins, not because of the sacrifice of animals, but because of the future sacrifice of the Lord Jesus, of whom the animal sacrifices were a picture:

> For the law having a shadow of good things to come, and not the very image of the things, can never with those sacrifices which they offered year by year continually make the comers thereunto perfect. In those sacrifices there is a remembrance again made of sins every year. For it is not possible that the blood of bulls and of goats should take away sins. (Hebrews 10:1, 3-4)
> We are sanctified through the offering of the body of Jesus Christ **once for all**. (Hebrews 10:10)

Thus when the Lord was performing His earthly ministry, He both healed the sick and forgave sins on account of His future sacrifice upon the cross.

Note, too, that the Lord's earthly ministry took place before His death and resurrection: no healings are recorded after His resurrection and before His ascension. Consequently, in order for Matthew to show that Jesus was fulfilling Isaiah's prophesy, he has to relate it to some healings. Since these all happened before the crucifixion, these are the ones he uses.

It should also be pointed out that the original context of the prophecy of healing in Isaiah is very much that of the cross.

When Peter quotes the phrase 'by whose stripes ye were healed', is this not in the context of enduring affliction, rather than avoiding it?

In I Peter 2, the Apostle is dealing with the subject of submitting to authority. From verse 18 he is exhorting slaves to submit to their masters, enduring with patience any hardship they might suffer. There is a strong indication that these hardships include beatings:

> For what glory is it, if, when ye be buffeted for your faults, ye shall take it patiently? but if, when ye do well, and suffer for it, ye take it patiently, this is acceptable with God. (I Peter 2:20)

Peter, then gives Christ as an example for them to follow, who,

> when he was reviled, reviled not again; when he suffered, he threatened not; but committed himself to him that judgeth righteously: Who his own self bare our sins in his own body on the tree, that we, being dead to sins, should live unto righteousness: by whose stripes ye were healed. (I Peter 2:23-24)

Some may argue that, since the passage is referring to enduring affliction, the phrase 'by whose stripes ye were healed' cannot refer to physical healing: they would say that Peter is arguing that Christians should endure suffering including sickness, and not seek to be healed from it. They would therefore say that the healing referred to is spiritual healing, being saved from sin.

Elsewhere[22] in this book it has been shown that there is a difference between affliction and suffering: we are called to suffer for the Lord, to endure affliction, including at times physical beatings; we are never, however, called to endure physical sickness. In scripture, sickness is always something from which we are to be delivered; it is a sign that something is wrong with us and should be dealt with. We found in the case of Paul that it was not a sickness that God would not remove but a demon sent 'to buffet' him: it was physical suffering but not sickness. It is interesting that here Peter uses the same Greek word, *to buffet,* to describe the afflictions a slave may suffer. It does not, however, describe sickness.

It has also been shown that physical healing and spiritual healing go together – that they are two sides of the same thing, with the physical body manifesting what is happening in the spirit. So when Peter refers to healing, he means both physical and spiritual at the same time. The slaves were therefore given an encouragement to suffer patiently as Christ did, perhaps with the hope that through their behaviour they will win their masters over to the Lord. As they received their spiritual and physical healing on account of Christ's stripes, perhaps their masters will be won as they see them receive stripes of their own without complaint.

---

[22] *See* What about injury, *page 48, and* Paul's thorn in the flesh, *page 27.*

SECTION II
Guidance Notes

Faithful are the wounds of a friend.
(Proverbs 27:6)

Introduction

This section provides a guide to numerous different illnesses and their spiritual causes. Obviously a book of this type would have difficulty in covering every known disease. However, there should be sufficient information given to enable the individual to gain a basic understanding of the cause of his illness, even if the specific illness is not mentioned. All the major parts of the body are covered, as well as their major diseases. By understanding the basic principles of the relationship between sin and sickness, together with the symbolic relevance of each part of the body and each type of illness and symptom, a fairly accurate picture of the spiritual problem should emerge.

As stated at the very bottom of page 68, the individual needs to have the guidance of the Holy Spirit for a full revelation of their personal problem, so the importance of spending time seeking the face of God cannot be emphasised too strongly. The guidance in this section of the book will point the person in the right direction, but they will need final clarification as to their particular situation from the Lord.

It should also be pointed out that if a person seeks the Lord as to the cause of their illness, He will of course reveal it to them with or without the use of these notes. This book, however, serves to show that there is logic in every illness we receive and that there is information in Scripture as to the cause of illnesses.

Theory of connection

In determining the connection between a physical illness and its spiritual cause, there are three main factors. First is **the Bible**. In numerous passages, parts of the body are shown to represent a part of our spiritual make-up, for example, the heart, the bowels and the tongue. The context in which these terms are used will help to reveal their significance. Secondly, the connection between parts of the body and their spiritual counterparts can be understood with a degree of **logic**. If *blood* represents a person's life (see Leviticus 17:11) and the heart drives the blood round the body, then the spiritual heart is that which drives a person's life. Thirdly and most importantly, **the Holy Spirit** gives revelation and shows, in combination with the Bible and logic, the causes of illnesses. These three are then tested and confirmed by observation and human experience.

This has been my method in discovering the causes of different illnesses, and the way the Holy Spirit has confirmed my conclusions has been breathtaking and extraordinary.

In determining the spiritual cause of illness, several other factors should be noted.

Degrees of illness
The seriousness of the illness will indicate the seriousness of the spiritual problem *for that particular person*. God deals with us as individuals and the chastisement is in relation to an individual's own situation, not in comparison with other people. For example, if God determines that it is very important for a person to be a good listener and they are falling short, they may become profoundly deaf, even though they are better at listening than many others. It is because it is a vital issue for that person.

Combination
In trying to determine a spiritual problem, it is necessary to bring together the different factors involved, namely, the part of the body affected and the symptoms. For example, a person may have dry, itchy hands. We learn three things from this: 1) The part of the body (the hands) tells us that the problem relates to the person's work. 2) Symptom A (the dryness) indicates that the person is not enjoying the work God has given them

to do. 3) Symptom B (itchiness) indicates the person wishes they were doing something else. Further complications indicate further developments. If the hands become so sore that they cease to function properly, it means that the attitude towards work is so bad that it is preventing the person from doing their work properly.

Right and Left
When dealing with parts of the body of which there are two, such as hands, eyes and ears, the position of the sick part of the body will have a bearing on the interpretation of the illness (*see* Right and Left, *page 118*).

Symbolism and remedy
Each illness has two features. First it symbolises the spiritual condition of the person. For example, a person who carries their spiritual burdens may get a bad back. The bad back slows them down, stops them from working effectively, and limits what they can do. This symbolises the fact that spiritually, through carrying their burdens, they have become slow, less effective, and limited. By casting their burdens on the Lord they can be released, and become fast-moving and more effective.

However, each illness also has a remedial effect: it should help the person to deal with the particular spiritual problem. If a person who carries his burdens gets a bad back, it should so limit him that he gets fed up, and ceases to worry about things.

How to use the reference section
The reference section contains both parts of the body and its own peculiar ailments, as well as specific diseases which may affect any part of the body, such as cancer. It will be found very valuable to read the whole section, not just the paragraph relating to your own illness. It will also be found helpful to read as much of the reference section as possible, in order to learn the way in which illnesses reveal spiritual problems.

When words are underlined it means that they are dealt with under their own heading. Please look them up in the index.

Quick Reference

A brief summary of illnesses, parts of the body and their spiritual meanings

It may at times be helpful to refer to this concise reference section for a quick explanation of an illness or part of the body, particularly when putting different factors side by side. Most of these topics are dealt with fully in the main reference section, so obviously the brief explanation of each term given here is somewhat inadequate.

Abscess – defensiveness regarding a sin
Ache – using a faculty in our own strength, trying too hard
Acid reflux – returning to things
Acne – pride
Addiction – idolatry
Adrenaline – excitement
Alcoholism – idolatry
Allergies – inappropriate thoughts & associations
Alopecia   lack of personal glory
Alzheimer's – failing to retain God in the mind
Anaemia – lack of vitality due to inadequate spiritual fellowship
Angina – small-mindedness, meanness
Anorexia nervosa – trust in self rather than God
Aphasia – lack of care in conveying/apprehending meaning
Apocrine glands – how one's emotions appear to others
Appendicitis – lack of conscience with regard to attitude towards others
Appetite – spiritual appetite, for work, fellowship, Word of God
Arm – strength and power in one's work
Arrhythmias – driving one's life to the wrong rhythm
Arthritis – bitterness towards others
Asthma – constraining the Holy Spirit
Autism – complacency arising from self-sufficiency
Back – where burdens are carried
Bacteria – attack of the Enemy
Bad Breath – offensive speech
Barrenness – spiritual barrenness

Bladder – desire to express emotion

Blood – life

Blood circulation – whether *life* gets to areas of your existence

Blushing – overheating regarding how one is seen

Bone marrow – soul/character/personality

Bones – family

Breast – children (offspring)

Bulimia nervosa – conflicting self-love

Cancer – a sin eating away at one's person

Candida – lack of love/desire for other people

Cerebral palsy – lack of control over areas of life/actions

Chicken pox – pride in response to sins of others

Cleft lip/palate – incomplete divide between thought and word

Cluttering – lack of focus in conveying meaning

Coldness – spiritual coldness, lack of warmth towards others, lack of passion (Revelation 3:15)

Colds – fleshliness occurring from overwork

Congenital disorders – dominant hereditary trait that needs correcting

Constipation – lack of mercy

Coronary thrombosis – small-mindedness blocking flow of life to the heart

Cramp – restrictive attitude in an area of one's life

Cystic fibrosis – lack of grace

Cystic tumour – something pointless growing in one's life

Depression – uncrucified self

Diabetes – not regulating the amount of pleasure/tolerance in one's life

Diaphragm – inner strength, resolve and decisiveness

Diarrhoea – not seeing the value of other people

Digestive system – attitude towards other people

Dilated cardiomyopathy – being too big-hearted, all-embracing

Down's Syndrome – pride and complacency from personal excellence

Dry skin – lack of joy/enjoyment

Dumbness – inappropriate use of the voice

Dyslexia – lack of care in conveying/apprehending meaning in writing

Dyspraxia – not being careful about actions

Dwarfism – being big in one's own eyes (therefore small)

Ears – spiritual hearing

Eating disorders – *see under individual types*
Eccrine glands – talking about areas of one's life
Eczema – lack of joy
Egg – idea, plan
Embolism – restrictive attitude which affects other areas of one's life
Encephalitis – mind being misused
Endocarditis – spiritual heart affected by a particular sin
Endocrine – instincts
Epilepsy – pride of life, intellectual pride
Eyes – spiritual vision
Fat, oil – enjoyment, pleasure, joy (Isaiah 61:3; Psalm 45:7)
Fatigue – lack of spiritual rest
Feeling, sense of – spiritual feeling
Feet – associations/the spiritual walk/where one places one's trust
Fever – becoming overheated
Flatulence – vain talking, doubting over food
Food intolerances – not enjoying the fellowship of certain people
Fragile Skin – being easily offended
Gall – discretion
Growth – same as *tumour*
Growth hormone – feeling the need to grow, improve, do more
Haemorrhoids – losing sight of grace
Haemophilia – wasting life
Halitosis – offensive speech
Hallux valgus – being overbearing towards associates
Hand – relates to work
Hardened arteries – unbending attitude, hard heartedness
Head – relates to authority
Heart – one's drive in life
Heart Attack – spiritual heart partially ceases to function
Heart failure – spiritual heart fails through fear
Heat – spiritual heat/passion (Revelation 3:15)
Hernia – moving out of one's sphere of service
Herpes – lack of care about an area of one's life
Hip – submission to God, defining point in one's life
HIV/AIDS – lack of conscience
Hole in the heart:
   a. Right to left shunt – trying to drive one's life without God
   b. Left to right shunt – spending too much time preparing to live rather than living.

Homosexuality – vanity, self love

Hormone – instincts

Hydrocephalus – intelligent thought not turned into action

Hyperthyroidism – excessive zeal

Hypertrophic cardiomyopathy – being excessively strong-willed

Hypothyroidism – lack of faith

IBS – irritable attitude towards others

Immune system – conscience

Impotence – a man submitting to a woman

Incontinence – excessive unnecessary confession of sin

Infectious diseases – sin caused by one's response to the sins of other people

Inflammation – indicates part of the soul is infected with sin, and much of the person's life is being directed and focussed upon sorting out this one thing

Insomnia – restlessness

Iron – strength

Itching – discontent

Kidneys – one's spiritual reins, the things that guide one's life

Knee – relates to strength (which comes from prayer)

Labour pains – relates to holiness

Left – *see* Right and Left

Legs – a person's strength in standing and moving spiritually

Leprosy – pride which affects one's reason

Lips – relates to one's words

Liver – honour

Long-sightedness – focussing only on the big picture and the future, not the immediate

Loss of appetite – lack of appetite for work, life and fellowship

Lungs – response to the inner working of the Holy Spirit

ME – lack of spiritual rest

Measles – sinning as a result of the person's response to the words of another person

Meningitis – not respecting/protecting one's mind

Menorrhoea – wasting life through not being focussing energies on one's children

Menstrual pains – lack of holiness

Mental illness – idolatry (*see also* Depression)

Miscarriage – idolising one's children

Motor Neurone Disease – failing to control different areas of one's life
Mouth – relates to one's words
Multiple sclerosis – lack of enjoyment of life
Mumps – sinning as a result of the person's response to the words
    of another person
Muscle – spiritual strength
Nasal congestion – lack of spirituality/openness to the Holy Spirit
Neck – submission
Neurological – relates to use of mind
Neuron – decision
Nose – relates to spirituality
Obesity – big self-life
Oestrogens – female characteristics: nourishing, caring
Oil, fat – enjoyment, pleasure, joy (Isaiah 61:3; Psalm 45:7)
Overweight – big self-life
Pancreas – understanding
Parasite – allowing someone to take advantage of you
Parkinson's disease – lack of forward movement in the spiritual life
Pleural cavity – the things that surround one's spiritual life
Pleurisy – a problem in one's attitude towards spiritual things
Post nasal drip – contentiousness, flow of thoughts
Prostate – warmth, especially towards women
Rash – being overheated with regard how one is viewed
Respiratory – relates to being filled with the Holy Spirit
Right and Left – right refers to the more important issues in
    one's life, especially the spiritual things; left refers to the less
    important things in one's life, especially the temporal matters
Rubella – sinning as a result of the person's response to the words
    of another person
Saliva – words
Salt – grace (Colossians 4:6)
Senses – spiritual faculties
Sensitivity (e.g. teeth, ears) – oversensitivity in an area
Sepsis, Septicaemia – corrupt spiritual life/character
Shaking – fear
Shin – one's strength to stand
Shingles – pride in response to sins of others
Short-sightedness – inability to see the big picture and the future,
    focussing only on the immediate situation

Sinuses – openness to the Holy Spirit through an absence of other things, the necessary spiritual vacuum

Skin – how one appears to others and oneself, pride

Smallpox – pride in response to sins of others

Smell – perception

Sores – lack of care over an area of one's life

Speech impediment – inability to express meaning

Spleen – discernment

Squint – lack of single-mindedness

Stomach – one's response to events and conversations after they have occurred

Stroke – unconsecrated mind

Stutter – holding back from expressing oneself fully

Sweat – words

Taste – discernment

Teeth – attitude towards one's family, work

Testicular diseases – relates to one's attitude towards one's children, plans, or things produced

Testosterone – male characteristics: leadership, strength, authority

Thrombosis – flow of life blocked by small-mindedness

Thumb – one's leadership and direction in the realm of one's work

Thyroid – relates to faith and zeal

Tinnitus – listening to wrong voices, critical attitude, lack of love

Tongue – relates to words

Tonsils – conscience with regard to one's words

Trembling – fear

Tumour – something growing in one's life (either benign or harmful)

Ulcers – lack of care over an area of one's life

Underweight – trust in self rather than God

Urinary – relates to expression of emotion

Uterus – relates to launching children into the world, or bringing a plan into effect

Varicocele – applying too much life to children/a plan, idea

Venereal diseases – relate to sexual issues

Vocal problems – inappropriate use of voice

Vomiting – *see* acid reflux

Water – words

Weight problems – relate to attitude towards self

Wound – mistake, sin

Allergies

Spiritual cause: **an association with something improper**

Scriptures
- Wherefore come out from among them, and be ye separate, saith the Lord, and touch not the unclean thing; and I will receive you. (II Corinthians 6:17)

Explanation of connection
In physical terms, when we have an allergy, it means that the body deems certain things as unhelpful for its own wellbeing and reacts against them. It seeks to expel the allergen as quickly as possible. If we breathe in an allergen, we may sneeze; if we touch an allergen, our skin reacts, becoming red and itchy; if we eat an allergen, we may have diarrhoea, as our bowels try to flush it through our system. Any of these reactions can have a further effect on the whole body.

In spiritual terms, an allergy indicates that we have something in our lives that needs to be expelled. These things may not be wrong in their own right, but they are inappropriate for us as individuals and at that particular time. Very often we are slow to detect the associations that are unhelpful to us spiritually. That's why the Lord gives us physical allergies to show us how we are being affected spiritually.

The different parts of the physical body which are affected by allergens have spiritual counterparts. When our breathing is affected, it means an inappropriate thought has entered into our minds and is affecting our being filled with the Spirit (*see also* Respiratory). People who suffer from various allergies which affect their breathing, such as hay fever, will be those who allow lots of strange thoughts and ideas to come into their minds. A brief moment of allergy will indicate a passing unchecked thought. Inappropriate thoughts would include both things that should never be thought about, as well as things that the Lord does not want us to consider at that particular moment. A person may be praying for something, but suddenly remember he needs to pay a bill. It is not wrong for him to think about paying the bill at an appropriate moment, but it is inappropriate just when he is praying. Equally, many Christians will suffer thoughts of condemnation and allow them to remain unchecked. Sneezing is a method by which our bodies quickly expel a foreign body from our respiratory system. This indicates that a thought should quickly be expelled from our minds. Helpfully, sneezing physically serves to distract our minds and stop our train of thoughts.

When our skin is affected, we are coming into contact with something inappropriate in our lives (*see also* Skin). This is more severe than an allergy that affects our breathing: we have moved from thinking to being actively involved with something.

When it is a food allergy, it means we are having fellowship in our lives with something that is harmful to us. When we have fellowship with someone it is food to us (*see introduction to* Digestive System). To have fellowship with other Christians is good food for us. However, to have fellowship with ungodly things, to go to pubs and night clubs, to watch television (so much of which is worldly or unclean), to read worldly or unclean books, is to eat something inappropriate for us; it is like eating at the table of devils.

> But I say, that the things which the Gentiles sacrifice, they sacrifice to devils, and not to God: and I would not that ye should have fellowship with devils. Ye cannot drink the cup of the Lord, and the cup of devils: ye cannot be partakers of the Lord's table, and of the table of devils. (I Corinthians 10:20-21)

God calls us to be separate from the world: not to be joined together with what is unrighteous or profane.

> Be ye not unequally yoked together with unbelievers: for what fellowship hath righteousness with unrighteousness? and what communion hath light with darkness? And what concord hath Christ with Belial? or what part hath he that believeth with an infidel? And what agreement hath the temple of God with idols? for ye are the temple of the living God; as God hath said, I will dwell in them, and walk in them; and I will be their God, and they shall be my people. Wherefore come out from among them, and be ye separate, saith the Lord, and touch not the unclean thing; and I will receive you. (II Corinthians 6:14-17)

Way of healing

Observe that you have inappropriate things in different areas of your life: you are thinking about things, or coming in contact with things, or having fellowship with things which are not appropriate for you as a Christian. Confess this to the Lord and turn from it and he will deliver you of your allergy.

Helpful scriptures

Philippians 4:8; Ephesians 5:1-13; 2 Corinthians 6:14-17

Alopecia

Spiritual cause: lack of personal glory, not caring how one appears to other people

Scriptures

- And the man whose hair is fallen off his head, he is bald; yet is he clean. And he that hath his hair fallen off from the part of his head toward his face, he is forehead bald: yet is he clean. (Leviticus 13:40-41)
- And they shall make themselves utterly bald for thee, and gird them with sackcloth, and they shall weep for thee with bitterness of heart and bitter wailing. (Ezekiel 27:31)
- Cut off thine hair, O Jerusalem, and cast it away, and take up a lamentation on high places [bare hilltops]; for the LORD hath rejected and forsaken the generation of his wrath. (Jeremiah 7:29)
- Doth not even nature itself teach you, that, if a man have long hair, it is a shame unto him? But if a woman have long hair, it is a glory to her. (I Corinthians 11:14-15)
- The hoary head is a crown of glory; It shall be found in the way of righteousness. (Proverbs 16:31 ASV)

Explanation of connection

Our hair is a natural crown of glory to us: it beautifies our appearance. A person who has a character that is glorious and attractive to other people will have a good head of hair. Thus, speaking of the Lord Jesus, Solomon says:

His head is as the most fine gold, his locks are bushy, and black as a raven. (Song of Solomon 5:11)

A person whose character and person lacks personal glory may suffer with alopecia. It must be understood that this does not refer to spirituality or spiritual glory and radiance, but to glory regarding the person's own character. A lack of personal glory is not sin – it just means the person does not make themselves appear personally attractive to others. They may, for example, be very blunt or dry in manner. This is not a sin, but it is not wholly necessary. A person can be spiritual without personal glory or unspiritual with personal glory. Thus Elisha was bald (II Kings 2) and though He was greatly used by God in blessing, he called down curses upon children who mocked him and could be very blunt in his dealings with people (II Kings 13:19; II Kings 5:27). Absolom, in contrast, wicked as he was, was hugely attractive and charismatic, stealing the hearts of his fellow-countrymen, and he had a tremendous head of hair. However, it is possible to be spiritual and be warm and attractive to others.

There are several reasons for a lack of personal glory.

First, a person may be so seeking after God, that they humble themselves, wanting every vestige of *self* to disappear. This may go with an ascetic lifestyle, as they deprive themselves of luxuries and comforts. Such a person will want only Christ to be seen and not themselves. This may cause them to have a dry character, though they may have a strong and close walk with the Lord. This may be seen particularly at times of repentance and deep contrition. However, in such cases, after humbling themselves before God, identifying with Christ in His death, they should emerge with a glorious new character. (We see a picture of this in the law of the Nazarite, who shaved off his hair at the start of a special time of holiness but then let it grow as a sign of his glorious purity, until the period of separation was fulfilled – see Numbers 6).

Secondly, you may not care how you appear to others – you may be blunt in your dealings with people.

Thirdly, a person may have a lack of enthusiasm, with no appetite for good things. Paul says to Timothy that the 'living God... giveth us richly all things to enjoy' (I Timothy 6:17). (*See also* Thyroid).

Fourthly, a person may have a shameful life, lusting after the things of this world and so bringing dishonour on themselves. Paul talks of people 'whose end is destruction, whose God is their belly, and whose glory is in their shame, who mind earthly things.' (Philippians 3:19)

Way of healing

Confess that your character has lacked personal glory and radiance: you have not made yourself attractive to others. Perhaps your character has become dry as you have ceased to enjoy the rich things that God has provided for us. Perhaps you are blunt in your dealings with other people, not caring how you come across. Alternatively, perhaps you have made yourself dishonourable through shameful behaviour. See that you have not just died with Christ but risen with Him and been glorified. As you gaze upon the one who is all-glorious, you have a crown of glory which you can continually cast at His feet.

Helpful scriptures
II Corinthians 3:18; I Corinthians 9:19-22;

Arthritis

Spiritual cause: bitter attitude towards others. This can be manifested in short-temperedness, envy etc.

Scriptures
- And not holding the Head, from which all the body by joints and bands having nourishment ministered, and knit together, increaseth with the increase of God. (Colossians 2:19)
- ...being knit together in love... (Colossians 2:2)
- Christ, From whom the whole body fitly joined together and compacted by that which every joint supplieth, according to the effectual working in the measure of every part, maketh increase of the body unto the edifying of itself in love (Ephesians 4:16)

- A sound heart is the life of the flesh: but envy the rottenness of the bones. (Proverbs 14:30)

Explanation of connection

As Christians we are described in the Bible as different parts of the body (I Corinthians 12:14-30). Some are hands, others eyes, others ears. All the parts of the body are connected to the rest of the body by joints of different kinds. When we have an abrasive attitude towards other parts of the body, it is like spiritual arthritis. It affects the other person, it affects us, and it affects the body as a whole.

You may have a wrong attitude towards other people. It may be bitterness, envy, a critical attitude, short-temperedness. You don't have an easy warm loving attitude towards everyone. You are not 'knit together in love' with other believers. It may be a bad attitude towards your husband or wife; it may be others in your family, or other people you know.

Way of healing

Think through your relationships with other people. Against whom do you have a wrong bitter attitude? Think of all examples, confess them to the Lord, and confess your bitter attitude as a whole. He will cleanse you and remove the arthritis.

Helpful scriptures

I Corinthians 12-13

Back, shoulders

Spiritual cause: Carrying your burdens/working in your own strength

Scriptures

- And it shall come to pass in that day, that his burden shall be taken away from off thy shoulder, and his yoke from off thy neck, and the yoke shall be destroyed because of the anointing. (Isaiah 10:27)
- And said unto the Levites that taught all Israel, which were holy unto the LORD, Put the holy ark in the house

which Solomon the son of David king of Israel did build; it
shall not be a burden upon your shoulders: (II Chronicles
35:3)
- For they bind heavy burdens and grievous to be borne, and
  lay them on men's shoulders; but they themselves will not
  move them with one of their fingers. (Matthew 23:4)
- I removed his shoulder from the burden: his hands were
  delivered from the pots. (Psalm 81:6)

Explanation of connection

In our lives there are various burdens that we may carry. A pastor
may feel the burden for the church he leads and feel it is up to him
to build the church. A father may carry the burden for his family,
in providing for them, looking after them, bringing up the children
well. Anything we have to do can be a burden, something that we
carry on our shoulders/backs. We can carry the burden of living the
Christian life.

However, the Lord does not call us to carry our burdens or to work
or live in our own strength. He speaks of 'casting all your care upon
Him; for he careth for you' (I Peter 5:7). The pastor does not have
to build the church: the Lord says that that is His work (Matthew
16:18). All He calls us to do is to **walk** with Him: to trust Him and
be obedient. That is the only yoke that He puts upon us.

Come unto me, all ye that labour and are heavy laden, and I will
give you rest. Take my yoke upon you, and learn of me; for I am
meek and lowly in heart: and ye shall find rest unto your souls.
For my yoke is easy, and my burden is light. (Matthew 11:28-30)

Way of healing

You've been trying to live and serve God in your own strength,
thinking that it's up to you to make things happen. Hand everything
over to the Lord. Allow Him to take care of everything. Confess to
Him how you have been carrying your own load: He will take your
burdens away and heal your back. All He calls you to do is walk
with Him.

Helpful scriptures

Psalm 55:22

Barrenness

Spiritual cause: **self-sufficiency/self-contentment**

Scriptures

- Sing, O barren, thou that didst not bear; break forth into singing, and cry aloud, thou that didst not travail with child: for more are the children of the desolate than the children of the married wife, saith the LORD. Enlarge the place of thy tent, and let them stretch forth the curtains of thine habitations: spare not, lengthen thy cords, and strengthen thy stakes; for thou shalt break forth on the right hand and on the left; and thy seed shall inherit the Gentiles, and make the desolate cities to be inhabited. Fear not; for thou shalt not be ashamed: neither be thou confounded; for thou shalt not be put to shame: for thou shalt forget the shame of thy youth, and shalt not remember the reproach of thy widowhood any more. For thy Maker is thine husband; the LORD of hosts is his name; and thy Redeemer the Holy One of Israel; the God of the whole earth shall he be called. (Isaiah 54:1-5)
- For it is written, Rejoice, thou barren that bearest not; break forth and cry, thou that travailest not: for the desolate hath many more children than she which hath an husband. (Galatians 4:27)

Explanation of connection

There is a principle in Scripture that those who say that they are self-sufficient are in fact barren. In the above passages, God says that the person who acknowledges that he has nothing, and makes God his provider, is fruitful. The one who says he has need of nothing is barren.

In the letter to the church at Laodicea, the Lord says to them that because they claim that they have in themselves everything they need and that they are self-sufficient, they really have nothing.

Because thou sayest, I am rich, and increased with goods, and have need of nothing; and knowest not that thou art wretched,

and miserable, and poor, and blind, and naked: I counsel thee
to buy of me gold tried in the fire, that thou mayest be rich;
and white raiment, that thou mayest be clothed, and that the
shame of thy nakedness do not appear; and anoint thine eyes
with eyesalve, that thou mayest see. (Revelation 3:17, 18)

If a married couple are barren physically, it means they are
seeking to meet their own needs in themselves and are therefore
spiritually barren: they are trying to be self-sufficient, to find
their own answers to their problems. Perhaps they try to find their
needs met in each other.

We see this in the case of Hannah and Elkanah in I Samuel 1.
Elkanah suggests that he is all that his wife needs, indicating that
this is their attitude in general. However, Hannah's barrenness
drives her to seek God and so she conceives. Similarly, Sarai
is unable to conceive a child with Abram, and their spiritual
barrenness is indicated by the fact that they try to remedy the
situation by their own means.

When God revealed His name to man, he declared Himself to
be 'I AM THAT I AM' (Exodus 3:14). That means that He is the
all-sufficient one. It is He therefore who is our provider and who
has everything that we need for our lives. He is the fountain of
water that never runs dry.

In Jeremiah 2, the Lord talks about His people seeking to
provide for themselves rather than coming to Him:

For my people have committed two evils; they have forsaken
me the fountain of living waters, and hewed them out cisterns,
broken cisterns, that can hold no water. (Jeremiah 2:13)

To try to meet our own needs in any area of our lives is to disregard
God. In Him is everything we need. Therefore, God wants us to
come to Him for everything.

How healing comes
You may have come to a place in your life where you feel self-
sufficient, that you can meet your own needs. You may feel that
your needs are met in your spouse, your work or your material
possessions. The Lord has made you barren to show you that

without Him you have nothing. He must be your continual source of life, your continual provider, whatever you have or don't have.

Confess to the Lord that you have been looking to yourself and to your spouse and not to Him for all you need, that you have become barren, and that without Him you have nothing. Once you have made Him your provider, He will provide you with a child.

Blood disorders

Spiritual meaning: relates to a person's life

Scriptures
- For the life of the flesh is in the blood. (Leviticus 17:11)

Explanation of connection
In scripture, blood represents a person's life. Therefore, the problem a person experiences with their blood speaks of their life (i.e. their spiritual life, the life within them).

Anaemia
In the physical condition, insufficient oxygen is reaching the person's body as a result of damage to or a shortage of red blood cells. This is because of deficiencies of iron, folic acid and vitamin B12 which come from an inadequate diet compared with the body's need, or an inability by the body to assimilate these nutrients (e.g. because of another illness being present). It may also be due to excessive blood loss (*see also* Haemophilia *and* Menorrhoea).

The spiritual parallel is that the Holy Spirit (the divine breath or oxygen) is not enlivening the whole being because of deficiencies in our spiritual diet/digestion. In order to be enlivened by the Holy Spirit we need a good diet of fellowship with God through prayer, reading the Bible and fellowship with other Christians.

Iron-Deficiency Anaemia
A lack of iron can in normal circumstances be cured by eating plenty of red meat. Children who are growing need extra iron, as do pregnant women, since they have a dependent child.

In spiritual terms, iron-deficiency anaemia means you are not getting enough strong meat. If you are to grow very quickly in spiritual things or if you need to minister to others in some way, you need a large amount.

> For when for the time ye ought to be teachers, ye have need that one teach you again which be the first principles of the oracles of God; and are become such as have need of milk, and not of strong meat. For every one that useth milk is unskilful in the word of righteousness: for he is a babe. But strong meat belongeth to them that are of full age, even those who by reason of use have their senses exercised to discern both good and evil. (Hebrews 5:12-14)

To eat strong spiritual meat is to have a strong encounter and relationship with the Lord Jesus Christ. Jesus said,

> Verily, verily, I say unto you, Except ye eat the flesh of the Son of man, and drink his blood, ye have no life in you. (John 6:53)

To feed on Jesus is to spend time in His presence getting to know Him, to dig deeply into His word, to have our lives taken up by Him. One of the main things that prevents us from feeding on Jesus is filling our lives and minds with things that are not really of God. In order to feed on Jesus we need to take our eyes off material possessions and the things of this world. We even need to ignore trivialities, including spiritual trivialities. We need to cut everything superfluous out of our spiritual experience and get down to a serious deep relationship with Jesus Christ. We need to be abiding in Him so that His life flows through us (John 15).

Anaemia as a result of blood-loss indicates a lack of spiritual strength because the person's life is being wasted in some way.

Pernicious Anaemia

This is due to a lack of vitamin B12 in the body, which in turn is caused either by a lack of meat or an inability to absorb it from meat that has been eaten.

In spiritual terms, the problem is either that you are not getting sufficient spiritual meat *(see notes for iron-deficiency above)* or that there is something preventing you from getting what you need from it. In the latter case, the cause may be that you are too restrictive in your spiritual outlook. You may be so keen to avoid error that you have discarded certain doctrines which are actually of God. You may have a restrictive circle of fellowship. You may be reading the Bible but not really having a full relationship with the Lord Jesus.

How healing comes
Confess that you have not really been feeding on Jesus and begin to enjoy a deep relationship with Him.

Haemophilia
In the physical condition, blood flows out of the body and does not stop. In the spiritual condition, the person's life is allowed to flow out through dissipation and nothing is done to check it. The fact that this is an hereditary illness indicates that it is an hereditary failing (*see also* <u>Congenital disorders</u>)

You allow your time and energy, your life in fact, to be wasted on trivia. You are pouring them away. You need to see that your life, your time and your energy, are precious, and should be used wisely for something worthwhile. Confess this to God and ask Him to heal you.

Menorrhoea
Since the uterus is the place where children are nourished and looked after before being launched into the world, menorrhoea indicates the woman is letting her life flow away rather than concentrating on the work of rearing children or preparing her children for life. She may, for example, be very busy doing useful things, but these may distract her from this essential work. Alternatively, she may have left the children somewhere else to be looked after while she concentrates on what she thinks is more important. In the case of a woman without children, it may also include wasting her life so that she is not in a position to have children.

See that the work of bringing up your children and getting them ready for life is a woman's highest calling. Devote your energies to that and let other things recede.

Narrowing of blood vessels

When this occurs the flow of blood in a vessel is restricted. In the spiritual, it means we are restricting the flow of life in some area of our lives; we are being small minded and mean-spirited in that area. We may be very narrow and restrictive in the area of our friendships, not letting them evolve and grow, or having a mean attitude towards our friends; or we may be restricting our marital or other family relationships, or our work life. In the case of **deep vein thrombosis**, it will indicate a sudden restrictive act or attitude.

Poor blood circulation

This occurs when we do not allow *the life/the life of God* fully to get to every area of our lives. We may enjoy our Christian service and put much energy into that, but may neglect our home-life. Alternatively we may not enjoy a full Christian social life.

Hypertension (high blood pressure)

Our blood pressure depends on two things: the force with which our heart pumps the blood and how wide or narrow the arteries are. If our heart pumps the blood too forcefully, this indicates that we are driving our lives at too hard a pace, and should rest in the Lord, doing only what He requires us to do. Narrowed arteries are dealt with above. When the two go together it means that we are trying to drive our lives very hard but that we are narrow-minded and restrictive in our approach to things. (*See also* <u>Angina</u>, *page 205*).

Varicose Veins

Varicose veins are large protruding veins on the legs which can be painful and uncomfortable. They come about because the veins which link the veins close to the skin (superficial veins) with deep veins (which transport blood back to the heart) have inefficient valves. Consequently, the superficial veins swell up with blood.

Varicose veins occur when we devote too much of our lives to superficial personal things and don't move on to deeper matters.

Embolism

An embolism is the obstruction of a blood vessel by a blood clot (or other particle of matter) which has travelled from another part of the body. This speaks of our lives being restricted in one area that then has an impact on another. For example, a person may have a bad attitude towards someone that they work with. This means they do not allow life to flow in the area of their work. As a result a blood clot may form in a blood vessel in the hand. It may then move to the lungs. This indicates that their restrictive attitude towards a fellow worker has an effect on their spiritual life.

Bones

Spiritual meaning: relationship to family

Scriptures
- And the rib, which the LORD God had taken from man, made he a woman, and brought her unto the man. And Adam said, This is now **bone of my bones**, and flesh of my flesh: she shall be called Woman, because she was taken out of Man. (Genesis 2:23)
- Then came all the tribes of Israel to David unto Hebron, and spake, saying, Behold, **we are thy bone** and thy flesh. (II Samuel 5:1)

Explanation of connection
When God made woman, He made her out of the rib of the man. His bones were then her bones, and her bones his bones. The same applies by extension to all of a person's family: children and parents are also 'bone of my bones'.

Bones therefore represent our relationship to and our role within our family. When a person's bones become diseased, it is an indication that their role within the family is not being carried out as it should. For example, a person who does not strongly support their family and play an active part may have weak bones. A person who tries to do too much for their family may have enlarged bones.

When David had sinned in the matter of Uriah the Hittite, Nathan told him that he would suffer in the sphere of his own family:

> Now therefore the sword shall never depart from thine house. (II Samuel 12:10)
> Because by this deed thou hast given great occasion to the enemies of the LORD to blaspheme, the child also that is born unto thee shall surely die. (II Samuel 12:14)

Thus, when David makes his penitential prayer in Psalm 51, he prays:

> Make me to hear joy and gladness; that the bones which thou hast broken may rejoice. (Psalm 51:8)

David is praying that he may see good in the fact that members of his own family will die. His actions had caused his family to suffer: his own broken bones demonstrated that his role within his family had not been carried out properly.

Bone diseases

Every person has a role to play in their own family according to their own gifts, abilities and position. Different failures to perform one's role correctly lead to different diseases of the bones. Whilst not every disease of the bone can be covered, some general principles may be observed.

- Bones that grow excessively indicate that the person's family has grown out of proportion in their mind. The person spends his life trying to support and help his family, carrying them as a burden the whole time. The person can think of nothing else. This may particularly happen when there are problems in the family, such as an errant spouse or family member. This includes both gigantism and acromegaly (*See also* Growth Hormone, *page 173*).

- If a bone starts to lose its blood supply and die, it may be that a person's relationship with their spouse/family is dying. It may come from lack of love, lack of time spent together.
- Weak and porous bones mean that the person is too weak in their role. They have ceased to exercise their proper function within the household. This could include not being active enough in supporting or watching out for the family. If one person lets others make all the decisions, they are failing to play their part and support the family. A wife, for example, has a role in advising her husband and helping him make decisions, pointing out where she feels he is going wrong, even though he has final authority in the household.
- Excessively dense bones may mean that the person has too dominant and strong an attitude towards their spouse/family. This may be a wife usurping authority or a husband being too dominant.

Seek the Lord in order to understand your wrong attitude regarding your family. Once you see it, simply confess it, and the blood of Jesus will cleanse you from all unrighteousness. You can then receive your healing.

Helpful scriptures
The role of men: I Timothy 3:4; I Peter 3:7; Titus 2:2, 6; Colossians 3:21
The role of women: Proverbs 31; I Timothy 5:10; Genesis 2:18; Titus 2:3-5; Ephesians 5:22
General: I Corinthians 7:10-16; I Corinthians 11:3; Ephesians: 5:22-33, 33; Titus 2:1-8

Bone marrow
- My soul shall be satisfied as with marrow and fatness; and my mouth shall praise thee with joyful lips: when I remember thee upon my bed, and meditate on thee in the night watches. (Psalm 63:5-6)
- A sound heart is the life of the flesh: but envy the rottenness of the bones. (Proverbs 14:30)

- And not holding the Head, from which all the body by joints and bands having nourishment ministered, and knit together, increaseth with the increase of God. (Colossians 2:19)
- For the word of God is quick, and powerful, and sharper than any twoedged sword, piercing even to the dividing asunder of soul and spirit, and of the joints and marrow, and is a discerner of the thoughts and intents of the heart. (Hebrews 4:12)
- *See also* Psalm 109:17-18

Bone marrow is the soft fatty tissue found in bones where most blood cells are produced. Oil/fat represents joy and blood represents life *(see pages 118 and 129)*.

There is a part of a person's being where joy is found, where the person's character or personality exists, the seat of a person's creativeness. This is the soul. It is the essence of the person, it is the personality.

When we have fellowship with other people and with God, we feed on the character of the other person and they feed on ours. We enjoy something of each other's personality. This is like the bone marrow supplying blood cells for the benefit of the rest of the body. Thus Paul says,

Christ, from whom the whole body fitly joined together and compacted by that which every joint supplieth, according to the effectual working in the measure of every part, maketh increase of the body unto the edifying of itself in love. (Ephesians 4:16)

When a person's bone marrow ceases to function and produce blood cells as it ought, it is an indication that the person's soul is not being productive. That means not being creative and fruitful, producing expressions of their character, demonstrations of their personality that can edify other people.

It is where two bones touch, at the joint, that they interact, but it is the marrow which produces blood cells which nourishes the rest of the body. So our soul is the place where characteristics are produced, and it is through interaction of our spirits, when we come in contact with one another, that we have fellowship together. We see this when Paul says,

> For the word of God is quick, and powerful, and sharper than any twoedged sword, piercing even to the **dividing asunder of soul and spirit, and of the joints and marrow**... (Hebrews 4:12)

Paul is adopting the rhetorical figure called a *chiasmus* which links together the first word with the fourth, and the second with the third, following the pattern 1-2-2-1: soul-*spirit-joints*-marrow.

In order to produce blood cells effectively, the bone marrow needs the nutrients necessary. This comes from having a good rich balanced diet, including sources of iron and vitamins. In order for a person's soul to be healthy and productive, a good spiritual diet is necessary. This means having plenty of fellowship with Christ and with other believers. A description of feeding on fellowship with God and other believers is found in Isaiah 25:6.

> And in this mountain shall the LORD of hosts make unto all people a feast of fat things, a feast of wines on the lees, **of fat things full of marrow**, of wines on the lees well refined. (Isaiah 25:6)

It is necessary to spend good time in the presence of the Lord Jesus, reading the Bible and communing with Him, and then to spend time enjoying the company and fellowship of other Christians. (*See also* <u>Digestive System</u> *for more information on the spiritual diet).*

Way of healing
Confess that you soul has become dry, and that this has come from not enjoying the fellowship of God and of other Christians. See that God made you to be fruitful, and ask for your healing.

Helpful Scriptures
John 6 (especially verses 48-65); Colossians 1:9-10

Breast

Spiritual meaning: **attitude towards one's children**

Scriptures

- Rejoice for joy with her, all ye that mourn for her: that ye may suck, and be satisfied with the breasts of her consolations; that ye may milk out, and be delighted with the abundance of her glory. For thus saith the LORD, Behold, I will extend peace to her like a river, and the glory of the Gentiles like a flowing stream: then shall ye suck, ye shall be borne upon her sides, and be dandled upon her knees. As one whom his mother comforteth, so will I comfort you; and ye shall be comforted in Jerusalem. (Isaiah 66:10-13)
- Ezekiel 23 (*the whole chapter should be read*)
- Even the sea monsters draw out the breast, they give suck to their young ones: the daughter of my people is become cruel, like the ostriches in the wilderness. The tongue of the sucking child cleaveth to the roof of his mouth for thirst: the young children ask bread, and no man breaketh it unto them. (Lamentations 4:3, 4)

Inasmuch as the breasts are used to nourish children, it follows that a wrong attitude towards one's children will be demonstrated with diseases of the breast, most notably breast cancer.

In Ezekiel 23 it speaks of a woman with children sacrificing them for various reasons. Three themes recur throughout the long chapter: 1) idolatry; 2) the sacrificing of children; 3) the bruising, wounding, and even the removal of breasts. In this chapter, the pattern is that a woman has children, becomes more interested in her lovers and other idols than her children and sacrifices her children to the idols. In many cases, it is her lovers that kill her own children.

The practical application

As a mother, you may feel that you love your children, may enjoy 'having' them, but your actions and real heart may indicate something different.

You may put your career before your children, preferring to go to work rather than look after them. You may put your own desires and preferences before the good of your children. Your relationship with your husband may be poor, perhaps leading to divorce and all the ill effects that that has upon children. You may run after different men, having numerous sexual partners, and making your children suffer as a result. Your new lovers may hate your children and abuse them, yet you choose to stay with the new man rather than caring for your children.

You may be sacrificing your children to other idols: the idol of educational ambition, caring more for the child's achievements than for the child itself. You may be showing a lack of love by not disciplining your children properly: for the sake of an easy life, you let them have their own way rather correcting them and punishing them fairly. Alternatively, you may 'do' everything right, but show a lack of love in what you say.

You may even have killed your own children before they were born through abortion, putting your career or your convenience ahead of the lives of your children. (Please see also the graphs relating abortions and breast cancer on page 39.)

In each case, as in Ezekiel 23, you have chosen to sacrifice your children for the sake of an idol, whether it be yourself, your career, another person, ambition or education.

When a man suffers from breast cancer it means that he is failing in this role of nurturing and caring for his children. The fact that the cancer is predominantly found in women emphasises the fact that it is predominantly their role to raise children.

How healing comes
See what idols you have had in your life, and how they have led you to fail to love your children. Simply confessing your sin before God and turning from it brings entire forgiveness, cleansing and physical healing.

You may have had an abortion long ago and never acknowledged it was wrong. Confess it before the Lord and you are utterly cleansed from it, as if it never happened.

Helpful Scriptures
Titus 2:4; II Corinthians 12:14; 1 Thessalonians 2:5-12; I Corinthians 13

Cancer

Spiritual cause: When a sin is allowed to grow

Scriptures
- ...And thou mourn at the last, when thy flesh and thy body are consumed, and say, How have I hated instruction, and my heart despised reproof; and have not obeyed the voice of my teachers, nor inclined mine ear to them that instructed me! (Proverbs 5:11- 13)

Explanation of connection
When the Lord wants to deal with a sin in our lives, he may allow an illness to come on the relevant part of our body in order to help reveal this to us. This is a form of God's instruction, His teaching. He will also speak to us in many other ways: through the Bible, through sermons, through our friends and family.

Very often we fail to listen and to deal with the sin. As time goes on, the sin grows in size, becomes more of a problem and starts to cat away at our lives. In the physical, this often shows itself as cancer.

We start with an illness in one part of our body indicating our sin. When the sin is not dealt with, the illness becomes worse. Eventually it becomes cancerous and starts eating away at our flesh. There then comes a stage at which the sin consumes our whole lives and the cancer takes over our whole body. If at this stage the sin is not dealt with, the person inevitably dies.

Way of healing
The place where the cancer started should indicate the root to the problem, the sin that has led to the cancer. If this does not clearly provide the answer, a careful seeking of the Lord and deep searching of the heart will reveal what is wrong. Whatever the sin, the Holy Spirit knows and He can reveal this to you. Make use of the excerpt from Finney on page 92.

Helpful scriptures
Proverbs 14:12, Amos 4:5-8; Isaiah 55:6-7; Jeremiah 33:3

Congenital disorders

Spiritual cause – dominant hereditary trait that needs correcting

Scriptures
- I the LORD thy God am a jealous God, visiting the iniquity of the fathers upon the children unto the third and fourth generation of them that hate me. (Exodus 20:5)
- This is the rejoicing city that dwelt carelessly, that said in her heart, I am, and there is none beside me: how is she become a desolation, a place for beasts to lie down in! every one that passeth by her shall hiss, and wag his hand. (Zepheniah 2:15)
- And thou saidst, I shall be a lady for ever: so that thou didst not lay these things to thy heart, neither didst remember the latter end of it. Therefore hear now this, thou that art given to pleasures, that dwellest carelessly, that sayest in thine heart, I am, and none else beside me; I shall not sit as a widow, neither shall I know the loss of children: but these two things shall come to thee in a moment in one day, the loss of children, and widowhood: they shall come upon thee in their perfection for the multitude of thy sorceries, and for the great abundance of thine enchantments. For thou hast trusted in thy wickedness: thou hast said, None seeth me. Thy wisdom and thy knowledge, it hath perverted thee; and thou hast said in thine heart, I am, and none else beside me. (Isaiah 47:7-10)

Explanation of connection
When parents have a sinful character trait that they are unaware of, or don't care about, they can very easily pass this on to their children. This will have serious consequences, because, if it is unchecked, each subsequent generation will be worse than the last, becoming more and more sinful in this regard. In order to prevent this from happening, God gives an illness that should help to reverse this effect and stop the spiritual degeneration of the family. Thus parents that are intellectually proud may have a child with learning difficulties. This should serve to humble the parents

and demonstrate the value of those with more limited intellectual ability. (*For further explanation, see also* What About Children?, *page 53*)

In each case, the child is born with the particular sinful disposition itself: it is not suffering for the sins of the parents, even though it has inherited the disposition from them. Even a child with learning difficulties will still have a natural propensity to spiritual pride, hence the need for the illness which stops them committing the sin. If they were to confess it, therefore, they would be healed.

In the case of each congenital or hereditary illness, the parents will be complacent about the particular sin which causes it. Thus, the child has to have the illness to help to stop his following into the same sin.

Way of healing
By discerning and confessing the hereditary sin which has caused the hereditary illness, the child can receive healing. This can be done by the parents or by the child itself when it is old enough.

Cystic fibrosis
Cystic fibrosis, in simplest terms, is caused by an inability of the body to allow salt to enter various cells.

Since *salt* symbolises *grace (see* Quick Reference, *page 114)*, this indicates a lack of grace in a person's life. The person may speak as if they are full of grace but their actions show otherwise. (*See also* <u>Digestive System</u> *for appropriate symptoms.*)

Down's Syndrome

Spiritual cause: **pride and complacency from personal excellence**

When a person is gifted – intelligent, capable and successful – they can easily rest in their own merit, becoming careless and complacent. They cease to feel their utter dependency upon God, because they realise their own natural intelligence and ability. This is like saying, 'I am, and none else beside me' (Isaiah 47:10). In fact, their success and intelligence has become a limitation: since it has caused them to cease to depend on God, their only true source of wisdom strength and blessing, they now lack (in spiritual terms) everything they thought they had.

When a child is born with Down's Syndrome, it has an extra chromosome. As a result of this, it suffers various limitations, particularly impairment in learning and physical growth. It is therefore prevented from making the mistake of its parents and trusting in its own abilities, for it has to depend upon others. Interestingly, children with Down's syndrome are usually very happy and affectionate.

The extra chromosome is equal to the parents' exceptional gifts; the limitations equal to the parents' spiritual limitations.

The consequence of the child's being born with Down's syndrome should be to cause the parents to recognise their own limitations and so depend upon God.

How healing comes
See that without God you have nothing, in spite of any gifts that you might possess. Confess that your success has made you careless and caused you to cease to recognise your utter dependency upon God. Ask for your cleansing and for healing.

Autism

Spiritual cause: **Complacency arising from self-sufficiency**

Explanation of connection
The word *autism* comes from the Greek word for *self*. The condition is so named because the person affected has difficulty relating to other people so is happier with themselves than with others. They have difficulty in sensing how other people are feeling and are content to be in their own world.

When a person (without autism) is content with their own world and their own company, when they are self-sufficient and self-satisfied, focusing on their own world rather than sensing the needs and feelings of others, this is a kind of spiritual autism. Because they are so wrapped up in their own world and own affairs, they are unable properly to relate to those around them. When a child is born with autism, it is an indication that the parents are more concerned with their own lives than the lives of others, that they are living in their own world. The child has inherited this disposition. The illness is corrective because both children and parents are forced to depend on others.

Way of healing
Confess that your satisfaction with your own life has caused you to focus on your own world rather than the needs of others.

Helpful scriptures
Philippians 2:4; I John 3:16

Principles for other illnesses
When a person considers themselves to be proficient in something, it means that they have ceased to rely on the Lord in that area. This means that they are in fact utterly lacking in that area. Consequently, a child may be born very deficient in that area to show the parents their own lack and to cause the child to make up the lack (by having to rely on God in that area).

Mental impairment
Parents that are mentally proud have ceased to trust God for their intellect. Having children with mental impairment will indicate this, and that the child has inherited this spiritual problem.

Dwarfism
When a person is born with dwarfism it indicates that the parents are very big in their own eyes, and that the child has inherited this trait. *(Further information may be found at Growth Hormone on page 173, even though not all dwarfism is connected to this hormone).*

Lack of growth in arms indicates with-holding your hand from doing good.

Behold, the LORD's hand is not shortened, that it cannot save. (Isaiah 59:1)

(*See* Hand and arm)

Depression

Spiritual cause: **uncrucified self**

Scriptures
- O wretched man that I am! who shall deliver me from the body of this death? I thank God through Jesus Christ our Lord. So then with the mind I myself serve the law of God; but with the flesh the law of sin. There is therefore now no condemnation to them which are in Christ Jesus, who walk not after the flesh, but after the Spirit. (Romans 7:24-8:1)

Explanation of connection
As humans we are born with a corrupt nature. It is naturally sinful and rebellious. It is always failing. There is nothing good in it at all. The Bible calls this nature *the flesh*.

For I know that in me (that is, in my flesh,) dwelleth no good thing: for to will is present with me; but how to perform that which is good I find not. For the good that I would I do not: but the evil which I would not, that I do. (Romans 7:18, 19)

The *flesh* means *human nature.* It is what we are naturally like. The flesh always wants to receive glory; it is always thinking about itself. Yet it is often at war with itself, because it never comes up to its own standards. It wishes it were better looking, cleverer. It looks back at the past and sees all its mistakes. The more it looks, the more it becomes depressed, because it seems a hopeless case – it is a rotten decaying nature. It looks at the current situation and the future, and sees that everything is hopeless for it now, and will be in the future.

When we became Christians, however, the old nature was killed. It was put to death.

> I am crucified with Christ: nevertheless I live; yet not I, but Christ liveth in me: and the life which I now live in the flesh I live by the faith of the Son of God, who loved me, and gave himself for me. (Galatians 2:20).

We are now set free from that old corrupt nature. That means that we are free from condemnation as long as 'we walk not after the flesh, but after the Spirit.' (Romans 7:24-8:1) Walking in the Spirit means that we have reckoned the old nature to be dead and are now living for God through the life and strength of the Lord Jesus.

> Reckon ye also yourselves to be dead indeed unto sin, but alive unto God through Jesus Christ our Lord. (Romans 6:11)

A dead man doesn't seek praise, he doesn't care what people think of him; he allows Christ to do everything through him, rather than doing things in his own strength. He is dead to self but alive to God. His own life has been replaced by the life of God.

You see if we have been crucified with Christ, our old self is dead. No-one can condemn it, because it is dead. You cannot condemn a dead man. Every time our hearts or the devil condemns us, we can say, 'Condemn away, I am dead and Christ now lives in me.' We no longer think or care about ourselves, because we have reckoned ourselves to be dead.[23]

The trouble comes when we allow the old nature to raise its ugly head. We start to walk after the flesh again. We start to think about ourselves, we worry, we try to live and work in our own strength. Our service begins and ends with ourselves. We come up with our own ideas of what to do, perform them in our own strength and then desire some kind of appreciation and glory for it. Unfortunately,

---

[23] It will be helpful in overcoming depression to recognise the role played by demons. A person suffering from depression is being condemned by the devil. Although we are delivered from this condemnation by dying to self as outlined above, recognising the work of the enemy is an important factor in getting free. *See also* Satan and demons, *page 80.*

because the flesh is a failure, we start to fail immediately. We then look at ourselves and feel depressed because we are so hopeless. But all we have to do is say again 'I am crucified with Christ: this old nature is dead and now it is Christ living in me with all His perfect victorious life' – then we are free from that old nature.

The Apostle Paul suffered with this problem. He said,

> O wretched man that I am! who shall deliver me from the body of this death? (Romans 7:24)

He wondered how he could be free from his old sinful corrupt failing nature. Then one day he saw it, as he describes in the next verse:

> I thank God through Jesus Christ our Lord. So then with the mind I myself serve the law of God; but with the flesh the law of sin. (Romans 7:25)

Way of healing

There is no way in which we can improve the old nature. It is always corrupt, hopeless and sinful, and always will be. But through the Lord's death on the cross, it has been put to death once and for all, and if we walk after the spirit (that is, living as men dead to self but alive to Christ) we are free from condemnation and the victorious life of Christ flows through us.

Confess that you have allowed the old self to be alive. You have been thinking about yourself, not reckoning yourself to be dead. You haven't lived as a dead man. Consequently, you have come under condemnation.

See that all the condemnation points at the old man who is now dead, and that your life as a Christian is not your life, but the life of Christ in you. Everything in your life is to come from Christ and be done in His strength and for His glory.

> For of him, and through him, and to him, are all things: to whom be glory for ever. Amen. (Romans 11:36)

Helpful scriptures

Colossians 3:3-5; John 12:24; Galatians 6:14; Hebrews 2:9; Romans 6:1-11; Romans 7 & 8.

Digestive system

Spiritual meaning: attitude towards other people

Scriptures – see below

Explanation of connection

The Bible makes it clear that, as Christians, our spiritual food is the Lord Jesus Christ himself. He said,

> I am the bread of life: he that cometh to me shall never hunger; and he that believeth on me shall never thirst. ...My flesh is meat indeed, and my blood is drink indeed. (John 6:35, 55)

There are two ways in which we feed upon Christ. One is by spending time in His presence through personal encounter. As we seek His face, pray and read the Bible, He imparts Himself to us. The other way is by spending time with other believers (see below). When we have a problem with our digestive system, it indicates a problem in the way we feed spiritually.

The main problems in our personal feeding on Christ, through time alone with Him, have to do with a lack of spiritual hunger, failing to spend proper time with Him, or filling our lives with and feeding on things other than Christ. More information on this aspect of spiritual feeding can be found under Appetite, Anaemia, and food allergies (under Allergies). However, since most digestive problems are caused by our relationship to other Christians, that is the area concentrated on in this section.

The body of Christ

The Bible says that the fellowship that we have with other Christians is like spiritual food to us.

> The bread which we break, is it not the fellowship of the body of Christ? For we being many are one bread, and one body: for we are all partakers of that one bread. (I Corinthians 10:16, 17)

The Lord Jesus has said that His body is given as food for us

(I Corinthians 11:24, John 6:53). As believers, we have become the body of Christ. Therefore, when we have fellowship with other Christians (the body of Christ, the church), we are feeding on Christ. Since as Christians we have all received the Bread of Life, that is, Jesus, we have now become bread for each other. By spending time having fellowship with other Christians we are spiritually fed.

When we develop bad attitudes towards other Christians, it affects our ability to enjoy fellowship with them. This means we are no longer able to enjoy our spiritual food.

Consequently, our physical digestive system becomes diseased to tell us there is a problem.

Since the body of Christ, the church, contains every single true believer throughout the world, if we have a bad attitude towards a part of it, our spiritual diet is affected. We may have a bad attitude towards people of certain denominations, people who praise God in a particular way, who have different ways of doing things from our own, whom we feel to be less spiritual than ourselves, who hold to doctrines we disagree with. However, the Bible says that every single part of the body is necessary and has been put there for a reason.

> But now hath God set the members every one of them in the body, as it hath pleased him. And if they were all one member, where were the body? But now are they many members, yet but one body. And the eye cannot say unto the hand, I have no need of thee: nor again the head to the feet, I have no need of you. Nay, much more those members of the body, which seem to be more feeble, are necessary. (I Corinthians 12:18-22)

Therefore, if we dismiss a part of the body, we are dismissing part of our spiritual food, a relevant vital part of the Lord's worldwide church. A bad attitude towards a single believer or a whole group of believers is a bad attitude towards the body of Christ.

It is important that we should have the correct attitude towards the rest of the body, because it is the body of Christ Himself. It is exceptionally precious.

There are various ways in which we can abuse the Lord's body, the church.

- Not seeing the need for and enjoying spending time with **all other believers.** Simply being with them, as individuals or as groups, is to enjoy spiritual food, regardless of any spiritual conversation or lack of it. We should actively desire and enjoy the company of all other Christians.
- Not seeing the needs of other Christians. We can easily be so caught up with our own spiritual walk that we forget that other people are at different stages. They may be unable to go at our pace. Therefore we should wait for them and go at their pace. To try and lead people on too quickly in spiritual things is a way of failing to care for them. (See Genesis 33:12-14; Romans 14)
- Not seeing that the body is made up of many members, and that every member of the body is important. Sometimes we think we can do everything ourselves, instead of letting and encouraging other people to help us. If we try to work without the help of others, we will end up doing other people's work rather than our own. As a result, we will find that the work as a whole suffers. This applies not only to other believers but also to other groups of Christians and churches. Every believer, every church, has its part to play. They are responsible before God for the work they are called to do, and only for that.
- Not playing the part that God has given us in the assembly. This means that other people are often forced to do our work, or the work does not get done. Everyone suffers as a consequence.

Discerning the Lord's body

Having established in I Corinthians 10 that we are fed by our fellowship with other Christians, Paul continues the subject in the next chapter. He describes the way in which the Lord Jesus ordained that we should eat our spiritual food.

The Lord Jesus the same night in which he was betrayed took bread: and when he had given thanks, he brake it, and said,

Take, eat: this is my body, which is broken for you: this do in remembrance of me. (I Corinthians 11:23, 24)

Of course this passage speaks to us on a number of levels. Most obviously it talks about the Lord's sacrificial death for us and the way in which we do the symbolic act of breaking bread and drinking wine as an assembly.

However, on another most important level, it is dealing with the fellowship that we have with one another, our spiritual meal together.

Let us look, therefore at the first Lord's Supper. The Lord Jesus has gathered His disciples together and they are spending time together in His presence. The Lord describes this time of fellowship as 'my body broken for you'. Amongst other things, the phrase 'broken for you' means 'provided for you, made available for you'. In that the church is His body, when we come together and have fellowship in His presence, enjoying each other's company, we are eating and enjoying His body. His church is provided for our spiritual nourishment, and it is a broken church, spread throughout the world.

Moreover, we see the specific way in which we have to come together. On that first occasion, as He teaches the manner in which we are to have fellowship together, the Lord Jesus is there, providing for His disciples, caring for them, putting them first. He is not thinking about Himself but about them. And all this on the very night in which He knows He is going to be betrayed.

We must remember also that earlier He has put a towel around Himself and washed the disciples' feet. It is all the more remarkable when we recall that Judas was amongst them – he was not excluded.

So the Lord says, when you come together, putting each other first as I have done, you are really remembering me, because this is how I do things. Moreover, He says that this is showing forth His death until He comes again (I Corinthians 11:26). Why is that? Because He laid down His life for us, and we are told to lay down our lives for the brethren (I John 3:16).

The problem in the church at Corinth is that they have not been doing this. There are divisions amongst them (I Corinthians 1:11-

13, 11:18), and so when they come together to eat their spiritual food, they cannot do it.

> When ye come together therefore into one place, this is not to eat [or you cannot eat] the Lord's supper. For in eating every one taketh before other his own supper: and one is hungry, and another is drunken. (I Corinthians 11:20, 21)

In putting themselves first, Paul says they are preventing themselves from eating the Lord's Supper, enjoying fellowship together. Each one seeks his own food, rather than caring for the needs of others. They behave in ways that are disrespectful to the others there.

Paul goes on to say that 'whosoever shall eat this bread, and drink this cup of the Lord, unworthily, shall be guilty of the body and blood of the Lord.' By this he means that anyone not treating the church properly is guilty of the very body and blood of the Lord Jesus, because the church is His body and He gave His blood to purchase it. Note that unworthily means 'in an unworthy manner', not 'being unworthy', which is true of all of us.

Paul goes on to speak about the serious consequences of not honouring the church.

> For he that eateth and drinketh unworthily, eateth and drinketh damnation to himself, not discerning the Lord's body. For this cause many are weak and sickly among you, and many sleep. (I Corinthians 11:29, 30)

He speaks of 'discerning the Lord's body.' To *discern* means to see something as it really is. Therefore, in failing to see that the church is the body of Christ, in failing to see that it is precious in every part and honouring it, we are dishonouring Christ Himself.[24]

Paul therefore tells them to be careful to examine themselves when they come together, that they have the right attitude to one

---

[24] Note, however, that he is not referring to dishonouring the bread and wine (for example, by failing to see that they represent the Lord's physical body and blood). This is Roman Catholic teaching. The whole context relates to our attitude towards other believers.

another, that they prefer others before themselves.

> But let a man examine himself, and so let him eat of that bread, and drink of that cup. For if we would judge ourselves, we should not be judged. But when we are judged, we are chastened of the Lord, that we should not be condemned with the world. (I Corinthians 11:28, 31, 32)

Paul sums up the teaching with the words,

> When ye come together to eat, tarry one for another. (I Corinthians 11:33)

By waiting on each other, we discern the Lord's body.

How healing comes

In our relationships with other believers, we can be like the Corinthian church: more interested in what we are getting out of it rather than being concerned that others are being fed and looked after, more interested in our own personal encounter with God rather than being interested in the other believers. The other believers are there for our spiritual food. If we don't enjoy being with them, if we have unloving attitudes towards them, we cannot enjoy our food. If we confess our sin, healing will come.

Let us look at some digestive problems in more detail.

Diarrhoea, food intolerances, including candida, Irritable Bowel Syndrome (IBS)

These illnesses indicate you are not enjoying the whole of the body of Christ. Just as your body is particular in what it will digest, you may have become very particular in which Christians you love, or esteem highly or spend time with. Remember, the whole Body has been provided for us and we must honour every true believer and every assembly of true believers.

Just as your physical body becomes weak and painful because you can't digest certain food, so your spiritual life is weakened and hurt because you are not enjoying the whole body of Christ.

For candida sufferers, just as you have a fungus which stops you being able to enjoy certain foods that you eat, so your lack of love for other believers is like a fungus which stops you enjoying fellowship with other Christians.

In II Chronicles it talks about Jehoram. He decided that he had no need for his brethren and so he killed them. The illness he gets is a disease of the bowels.

And there came a writing to him from Elijah the prophet, saying, Thus saith the LORD God of David thy father, Because thou hast not walked in the ways of Jehoshaphat thy father, nor in the ways of Asa king of Judah, But hast walked in the way of the kings of Israel, and hast made Judah and the inhabitants of Jerusalem to go a whoring, like to the whoredoms of the house of Ahab, and also hast slain thy brethren of thy father's house, which were better than thyself: behold, with a great plague will the LORD smite thy people, and thy children, and thy wives, and all thy goods: and thou shalt have great sickness by disease of thy bowels, until thy bowels fall out by reason of the sickness day by day. (II Chronicles 21:12-15)

Sometimes we may think we have no need for our brethren and kill them in our hearts and with our words. As a result of this we may get a diseased bowel.

Food intolerances of different types will indicate different types of people whose fellowship we do not appreciate. Lactose (milk sugar) intolerance speaks of a bad attitude towards one's parents.

Constipation

The physical symptom of constipation is that food remains in the intestine and is not released. The body seeks to draw more out of it than is available and will not release it.

In our relationships with other people, we may expect too much of them, and this may lead us to be unmerciful. When someone does something, we may criticize them for not doing it better; when someone makes a mistake, we may be hard on them.

It is one thing to be aware that something could have been done better: without noticing such things for our own benefit, we lower our own personal standards. It is another, however, to respond with an unloving unmerciful attitude towards the other person.

We need to be aware that people have different needs and abilities, that there are different factors in their lives and characters which have an effect upon what they do. We need to treat them with mercy and compassion.

> But whoso hath this world's good, and seeth his brother have need, and **shutteth up his bowels of compassion** from him, how dwelleth the love of God in him? (I John 3:17)

Although John here is specifically speaking about showing a lack of compassion by failing to give to those in need, the principle applies to every lack of compassion and mercy.

Acid reflux, vomiting

When we have acid reflux, the contents of our stomach starts going back up the oesophagus. Vomiting is an extreme type of this. We are not always aware that we have acid reflux, because small amounts of acid can come up the oesophagus relatively unnoticed. It can be indicated by heartburn, a frog in the throat, sinusitis or by a sore burning sensation in the throat.

There are several particular spiritual causes of this, each of them to do with 'returning'.

Returning to old sins and returning to the past
- As a dog returneth to his vomit, so a fool returneth to his folly. (Proverbs 26:11)

When we return to sins of the past, it is like bringing up food we have already swallowed. Consequently we get acid reflux, or in extreme cases vomiting. To bring things up from the past in conversation has the same effect: we are seeking to devour things that we should have swallowed long ago. Often this may be someone else's mistakes of the past, or it may be our own. God says,

> Remember ye not the former things, neither consider the things of old. Behold, I will do a new thing; now it shall spring forth; shall ye not know it? (Isaiah 43:18, 19)

In that God always wants to give us something new, a fresh

revelation of Himself, it is wrong for us to be trying to eat yesterday's food. In Exodus 16, when the Lord gave the Israelites manna, they were instructed not to eat what they had collected the day before, but to collect and enjoy fresh manna every day. When they disobeyed God and tried to use yesterday's manna, they found that it 'bred worms, and stank' (Exodus 16:20). Of course, there are certain occasions when the Lord ordains that we should remember what He has done for us in the past, and to share testimony of this with others. However, we should be certain that it is God leading us to speak, that it is done in the spirit, not in the flesh.

Vacillating
- The LORD hath mingled a perverse spirit in the midst thereof: and they have caused Egypt to err in every work thereof, as a drunken man staggereth [lit: vacillates] in his vomit. (Isaiah 19:14)

When we vacillate, switching backwards and forwards from one opinion to the other, God says that it is like a man who is drunk, staggering this way and that. It is like vomit: having eaten, we bring it back up again.

When we feel we should do something and then change our mind, we are soon thrown into confusion. The more we think about it, the more we dither between the two opinions and the more confused we get. We end up like a drunken man in our confusion. Moreover, it is hard to extricate oneself once one has got entangled: the devil sees what is happening and ties us up more and more.

Vacillating can develop into a very bad habit and quickly affect your whole life. James says,

A double minded man is unstable in all his ways. (James 1:8)

However, in the preceding verses he also shows us how to be free from this problem.

If any of you lack wisdom, let him ask of God, that giveth to all men liberally, and upbraideth not; and it shall be given him. But let him ask in faith, nothing wavering. For he that wavereth is like a wave of the sea driven with the wind and tossed. For let not that man think that he shall receive any thing of the Lord. (James 1:5-7)

Deep down, we really know the Lord's will in our situation: it is often the thing we least want to do, the hard thing to do. In order to break free from the spin of indecision, we have to admit that 'The heart is deceitful above all things' (Jeremiah 17:9): our hearts can fool us. We then need to be filled with wisdom. We receive this by regaining our understanding of who God is.

> The fear of the LORD is the beginning of wisdom. (Psalm 111:10)

If we come to God and really want wisdom, He will give it to us. We need to bring our thoughts into subjection, guiding our actions by the word of God, not by feelings, circumstances, coincidences or things that people say: we need to apply godly wisdom to our lives. If we apply the simple truths of the Word of God to our situation, we will quickly be set free.

How healing comes
Confess to the Lord how you vacillate in your life. Fear God and apply godly wisdom to your life. Learn to get the Lord's mind on situations and then be instantly obedient: this prevents constantly changing your mind.

Appendicitis
The appendix is a part of the large intestine which is covered in lymph glands and therefore is part of the immune system.

The immune system symbolises our conscience. Since the appendix is part of the bowels it symbolises our conscience with regard our attitude towards other people. Appendicitis indicates a sudden bad attitude towards another person, perhaps including anger and hatred, and the fact that we have no conscience about it.

Bowel cramp
A cramp is a restricting, a tightening of a muscle. When it occurs in the digestive system it means a mean, limiting, restrictive

attitude towards others. It may be a sudden narrowness in attitude towards people in general, or someone in particular.

> Ye are not straitened in us, but ye are straitened [lit: cramped] in your own bowels. (II Corinthians 6:12)

Flatulence

There are two particular causes of this.

a) <u>Vanity</u>

When we suffer from flatulence, our bodies are bloated, puffed up, with gas. The spiritual equivalent is to be puffed up with vanity and self importance. In various places in scripture it uses the phrase 'puffed up' to mean proud and vain.

> Let no man beguile you of your reward in a voluntary humility and worshipping of angels, intruding into those things which he hath not seen, vainly puffed up by his fleshly mind. (Colossians 2:18)
>
> Knowledge puffeth up, but charity edifieth. (I Corinthians 8:1)

The word used for being puffed up is also the word for flatulence.

When we are conceited, proud of our own cleverness, this very often comes out in our speech.

> ...they speak great swelling words of vanity. (II Peter 2:18)

Instead of our conversation being edifying, something solid to build people up, it is empty and without value. It may be excessively witty, or we may delight to show off our knowledge. Paul says:

> Be ye therefore followers of God, as dear children; and walk in love, as Christ also hath loved us, and hath given himself for us an offering and a sacrifice to God for a sweetsmelling savour. But fornication, and all uncleanness, or covetousness, let it not be once named among you, as becometh saints; neither filthiness, nor foolish talking, nor jesting, which are not convenient: but rather giving of thanks. For this ye know, that

no whoremonger, nor unclean person, nor covetous man, who is an idolater, hath any inheritance in the kingdom of Christ and of God. Let no man deceive you with vain words: for because of these things cometh the wrath of God upon the children of disobedience. (Ephesians 5:1-6)

Consequently, flatulence can be caused by speaking vain, foolish words.

Helpful Scriptures
I Corinthians 4:5-7; Romans 12

b) Doubt with regard to food (and fellowship)
If we are filled with doubts regarding the food we eat, always worried about what it will do to us and for us, it is like suspending the food in mid-air and filling ourselves with emptiness.

And seek not ye what ye shall eat, or what ye shall drink, neither be ye of **doubtful mind** (Luke 12:29)

The word translated *doubtful mind* also means to have wind rising from the stomach.
The same can apply to our fellowship with other people. If we are always doubting whom we should speak with, rather than getting on and enjoying fellowship with everyone, it is like filling ourselves with wind.
Therefore, doubt regarding food and fellowship can cause flatulence.

Helpful scriptures
Philippians 4:6, 7, Luke 12:22-34

Food Allergies – *see under* **Allergies**

Gall – discretion
Gall, or bile, is a bitter digestive fluid secreted by the liver which aids digestion by breaking up fats. It also serves to neutralize acid from the stomach.
In spiritual terms, we need an element in our characters which

can deal with praise and honour when it comes our way so that we do not become over-pleased with ourselves. We might term this *discretion*. It is a kind of bitterness in us that responds with sense and realism when something good happens to us, to stop us becoming over-excited and carried away. It is a kind of dryness of attitude which can see the futility of things that are without value and brings realism into our situation. Equally, when we have sour feelings, such as from envy or from remembering former experiences, our discretion needs to deal with them, by showing us how futile they are.

When gall is mentioned in the Bible, it comes when people are showing a lack of discretion, generally through complacency. When Job was in a position of prosperity, then it was that he says that his gall poured upon the ground.

> I was at ease [careless], but he hath broken me asunder: he hath also taken me by my neck, and shaken me to pieces, and set me up for his mark. His archers compass me round about, he cleaveth my reins asunder, and doth not spare; he poureth out my gall upon the ground. (Job 16:12, 13. *See also* Jeremiah 8:7-14; Job 20:12-14)

Gallstones come largely because of a lack of full emptying of the gall bladder, or because the gall is not properly constituted. Gallstones will indicate a lack of exercise of discretion. A diseased gall-bladder will indicate that the faculty of discretion has become impaired in some way. An excess of gall will mean an excessively bitter character in relationships with other people (*see* Acts 8:23).

Way of healing
See that you need an element in your character which looks at things realistically, an antidote to euphoria and excessive excitement, a slight bitterness and dryness. See also that an excessively acerbic attitude is as wrong as excessive levity. Confess your failing and ask for your healing.

Helpful Scriptures
Luke 10:20

Pancreas (including cause of diabetes) – understanding

- But the fig tree said unto them, Should I forsake my sweetness, and my good fruit, and go to be promoted over the trees? (Judges 9:11)

The pancreas has two main functions: producing enzymes that help to digest food and producing hormones that control blood sugar levels.

In spiritual terms, this speaks of our *understanding*. Our understanding enables us to enjoy a deep relationship with someone: it enables us to digest our spiritual food. Our understanding also determines how much 'sweetness' we allow in our lives. If we are too nice and lenient towards people, embracing everything and not being sufficiently straightforward, we are showing a lack of understanding. This comes from a desire for an easy pleasurable life

A person with a diseased pancreas is not exercising their understanding. Diabetes indicates the person is too sweet – too tolerant and all-embracing; they will not be direct and deal with the harder things in life.

Stomach (*see also* peptic ulcer *under* Ulcers)

- And he said unto me, Son of man, cause thy belly to eat, and fill thy bowels with this roll that I give thee. Then did I eat it; and it was in my mouth as honey for sweetness. So the spirit lifted me up, and took me away, and I went in bitterness, in the heat of my spirit; but the hand of the LORD was strong upon me. (Ezekiel 3:3, 14)
- The righteous eateth to the satisfying of his soul: but the belly of the wicked shall want. (Proverbs 13:25)
- The words of a talebearer are as wounds, and they go down into the innermost parts of the belly. (Proverbs 18:8)

The stomach is the first place of digestion after the mouth, and its function is to break up large molecules into smaller ones. It is a holding place for food before it continues into the small intestine. After we eat, it should be the place where we feel satisfaction and contentment.

In spiritual terms, this speaks of our response to things, the way we digest situations and conversations after we have come across them/taken part in them. When we trust in God to take care of the situation, we will be left with a sense of peace and contentment. If we do not trust God, we will be worried and knotted up.

Stomach problems, therefore, indicate worry and lack of rest and contentment about things. They may also indicate critical attitudes after we have spoken to people or had contact with them.

Way of healing
When we worry, we are saying that we don't trust God, that we don't believe that He will look after things. Confess this, and ask for your healing.

Helpful Scriptures
Philippians 4:6-7

Dysphasia, aphasia

Spiritual cause: Lack of attention paid to conveying/ apprehending meaning

Scriptures
- Take heed therefore how ye hear: for whosoever hath, to him shall be given; and whosoever hath not, from him shall be taken even that which he seemeth to have. (Luke 8:18)

Explanation of connection
Aphasia is the term for a defect of the brain which removes a person's ability to communicate. Dysphasia is an impairment of this ability. The condition exists in spite of all the necessary factors for communication being in place, such as hearing, ability to make sounds, and normal intelligence. It is a kind of mental block. It may be evident in speaking, understanding speech, reading and writing.

In each case it speaks of a person's lack of care either in conveying or apprehending meaning. When a person cannot physically utter the words they wish to say, it means that spiritually they are not able to clarify their thoughts and convey their meaning to other people. They may have lots of thoughts, but they are unable to bring them together and express them to other people. When a person cannot comprehend language, it means they cannot comprehend meaning, what people are actually saying. In each case this is due to lack of care and attention in comprehending/conveying meaning. (For example, a person who cannot understand language would be someone who did not pay careful attention to the meaning of what people said).

Dyslexia

A person with dyslexia has difficulty with reading and writing, in spite of normal intelligence. They will typically misread words, seeing words and letters in the wrong order.

This speaks of a lack of attention paid to the true meaning of the written word. We may, for example, read a portion of Scripture, and put our own ideas into it, basing our interpretation on what we have always thought or been told. This is instead of carefully observing what the Word says for itself. Someone with dyslexia is forced to read slowly and therefore carefully to try to gain the true meaning of the words.

Dyslexia is understandably also related to auditory perception, when a person does not pay proper attention to the spoken word.

Dyspraxia

Dyspraxia is a disorder which impairs the person's ability to begin, organise and perform actions. It means that when a person tries to do something, their body does not act quite in the way intended. It shows itself as clumsiness, a lack of co-ordination.

In spiritual terms, this speaks of a clumsiness in the spiritual walk and service. Typically a person will not be careful in what they do.

Way of healing

Confess that there has been a lack of care in a particular area of communication or action. See the importance of paying careful attention to conveying meaning in words and understanding meaning in words. In the case of dyspraxia, see the importance of being careful and precise in what you do.

Helpful scriptures
Psalm 39, Psalm 37:23

Ears

Spiritual meaning: **Listening**

Scriptures
- But I, as a deaf man, heard not. (Psalm 38:13)
- They are like the deaf adder that stoppeth her ear; which will not hearken to the voice of charmers, charming never so wisely. (Psalm 58:4, 5)

Explanation of connection
Our physical hearing is directly related to our spiritual hearing. If we do not listen to other people and we do not listen to God, we may find that our hearing becomes impaired.

It can be easy to develop bad habits when talking to people. We ask them a question, but as soon as they start to speak we switch off. When someone is speaking we may not pay close attention to what they are actually saying. We hear the words but we don't apprehend the real meaning. Consequently, we afterwards think they have said something different from what they have actually said.

One of the underlying causes of this is an inability to relate to other people, including a lack of empathy. If we are unable to see things from the other person's perspective, we will be unable to understand what they mean.

This can apply very much to preaching. We may have so many preconceptions that we read into the sermon our own ideas and thoughts, rather than listening to the actual words.

It can also apply to our relationship with God. We read the Bible, we spend time with God, but we may not properly listen to what He is saying; we are filled with our own thoughts and our own preconceptions.

It is vitally important for our relationships with other people and with God that we listen very carefully to what they are actually saying. A large part of this is patience: quietly waiting to hear what they are really saying, rather than becoming impatient and switching off before we have heard what they are saying. Very often, the reason we do not listen to others is because we are too busy thinking our own thoughts whilst they are speaking or because we talk too much. We are more interested in our thoughts and words than in theirs. Since water symbolises words (*see* **Quick Reference**), fluid in the ears will indicate this.

Often if we are a poor listener in one relationship, we will be a poor listener in all our relationships.

The people that you have most difficulty hearing are those that you listen to the least. It may be a parent, a child, a pastor: the fact that you don't pay attention is demonstrated by your loss of hearing. When only one ear is affected, it indicates we are not listening in one area of our lives (*see* Right and Left, *page 118*).

Physical deafness has a remedial effect in that it forces people to listen: they may have to lip-read, or to have things written down, or have something repeated. In all these ways, the words are impressed upon the consciousness of the individual.

Way of healing
Confess to the Lord that you don't listen, perhaps that you are impatient, reading into people's words your own thoughts. It may also be necessary to go to individuals and confess to them that you have not been listening to them properly.

Helpful scriptures
Romans 12:10

Tinnitus

Spiritual cause: **Listening to wrong voices, critical attitude**

Scriptures
- Though I speak with the tongues of men and of angels, and have not charity, I am become as sounding brass, or a tinkling cymbal. (1 Corinthians 13:1)

- There are, it may be, so many kinds of voices in the world, and none of them is without signification. (1 Corinthians 14:10)

Explanation of connection

Since our physical hearing speaks of spiritual hearing, a ringing in our ears, or tinnitus, indicates that we are listening to things that are not of God.

As we go about our lives, various thoughts come to our minds. Some will come from God, some will come from our fleshly nature, and some will come from the influence of demons.

I Corinthians 14:10 says,

> There are, it may be, so many kinds of voices in the world, and none of them is without signification. (I Corinthians 14:10)

Although there are many kinds of voices in the world, it is up to us which we choose to listen to. Some thoughts may be temptations and things to lead us away from God but others may be right and proper things to help us. Long-term tinnitus indicates we listen continually to thoughts that are not of God, a sudden ringing in the ears indicates we have done it momentarily and need to refocus our minds on the Lord.

It is not always easy to distinguish between the voice of the Lord and the lying voice of the Devil. However, with the help of the Bible under the direction of the Holy Spirit we are able to judge between the two. This is the exact method that the Lord Jesus used when He was tempted:

> And the devil said unto him, If thou be the Son of God, command this stone that it be made bread. And Jesus answered him, saying, It is written, That man shall not live by bread alone, but by every word of God. (Luke 4:3-4)

Each time that the Lord is tempted by the devil, He responds by quoting the word of God. When we are under a spiritual attack, it is not enough to go on feelings, even when we are filled with the Holy Spirit, as the Lord was: we have to depend upon Scripture, the revealed word of God.

One of the chief temptations that the devil will bring to our minds is to hate other people. Critical thoughts may come to us. God says that if we have a lack of love for other people, when we speak we will sound like a clanging gong or a tinkling cymbal.

> Though I speak with the tongues of men and of angels, and have not charity, I am become as sounding brass, or a tinkling cymbal. (1 Corinthians 13:1)

We will tend to sound strident and irritating, criticising and finding fault. We will be insensitive to other people.

Thus, when unloving critical thoughts come to our minds and we listen to them and don't dismiss them, we may get tinnitus: a sounding brass or a tinkling cymbal in our ears.

Way of healing
Observe that you listen to thoughts that are not from God: perhaps fleshly thoughts, temptations from the devil. Perhaps you allow critical thoughts to remain unchecked. Confess it to God, seek God to know His real voice, and receive your healing.

Helpful scriptures
James 4:7; Philippians 4:8; 1 Corinthians 4:7; II Corinthians 10:3-5.

Eating disorders

Anorexia nervosa

Scriptures
- And they shall eat up thine harvest, and thy bread, which thy sons and thy daughters should eat: they shall eat up thy flocks and thine herds: they shall eat up thy vines and thy fig trees: they shall impoverish thy fenced cities, wherein thou trustedst, with the sword. (Jeremiah 5:17)
- Ye have eaten the fruit of lies [lit.: emaciation, leanness of flesh]: because thou didst trust in thy way, in the multitude of thy mighty men. (Hosea 10:13)
- He that putteth his trust in the LORD shall be made fat. (Proverbs 28:25)

Spiritual cause: **trust in oneself rather than in God**

Explanation of connection

In the passage from Jeremiah quoted above, because Israel has trusted in her own strength rather than in the Lord, she is told that she will have no strength when the enemy comes to devour her. The enemy will eat up all her good produce. By trusting in the Lord, Israel would be protected from the attacks of the enemy and would be provided for continually.

When someone trusts in themselves, it is like trying to get nourishment from within themselves, like devouring their own flesh. They are, in effect, looking to themselves for strength and seeking to be nourished by their own strength. Consequently, they waste away.

A person with anorexia will typically have 'low self-esteem'. It is a good thing to have no high opinion of ourselves, but when having done that we continue to seek to find strength from within ourselves, we quickly waste away. The answer to anorexia is not to increase one's self-esteem, but to regard oneself as dead to self and to find one's life and help in God. Tozer says,

> The victorious Christian neither exalts nor downgrades himself. His interests have shifted from self to Christ. What he is or is not no longer concerns him. He believes that he has been crucified with Christ and he is not willing either to praise or deprecate such a man.[25]

Way of healing

You have been seeking to find a solution to your problems within yourself, trusting in yourself to get you through life. God calls you to put your trust in Him, and let Him care for you and provide for you. Confess this, and ask the Lord to meet your need.

Helpful scriptures

I Peter 5:6-11

---

[25] *Man – The Dwelling Place of God,* A. W. Tozer, Ch.18.

Bulimia nervosa

Spiritual cause: **conflicting self-love**

Scriptures
- Therefore also will I make thee sick in smiting thee, in making thee desolate because of thy sins. Thou shalt eat, but not be satisfied. (Micah 6:13:14)

Bulimia is a condition in which a person repeatedly eats excessively and then seeks to purge their body of the food. The purging may take various forms, including induced vomiting, taking laxatives and excessive exercise.

This indicates the person is split between a very high opinion of themselves and a very low opinion. First of all they have a high opinion and want to give themselves everything they want – they want to build themselves up with excessive food. Then immediately they see themselves as not living up to their own standards in looks, character and abilities. Therefore they want to purge themselves – to reduce themselves in size.

In both cases, the person is idolising themselves. Even when they see their inadequacies, they are idolising themselves because they want themselves to be better-looking/more talented. (The person who says, 'I hate myself because I'm so ugly' really means 'I love myself and wish I were better looking.' If they hated themselves they would be glad they were ugly).

God wants us to have neither a high nor low opinion of ourselves – He doesn't want us to think about ourselves. To focus on ourselves is to worship ourselves rather than to worship God (*see also the quotation from Tozer under* <u>Anorexia</u> *opposite. For a fuller treatment of this theme please see* <u>Obesity</u>. *See also* <u>Depression</u>.)

Way of healing
Confess that you have been loving yourself and made yourself your own idol. See that you need to be one dead to self but alive to God.

Helpful scriptures
Exodus 20:3

Loss of appetite (see also <u>Digestive System</u>)

Spiritual cause: lack appetite for God, His Word, or work (idleness)

Scriptures
- Man shall not live by bread alone, but by every word that proceedeth out of the mouth of God. (Matthew 4:4)
- Jesus said unto them, I am the bread of life. (John 6:35)
- Jesus saith unto them, My meat is to do the will of him that sent me, and to finish his work. (John 4:34)
- For even when we were with you, this we commanded you, that if any would not work, neither should he eat. For we hear that there are some which walk among you disorderly, working not at all, but are busybodies. Now them that are such we command and exhort by our Lord Jesus Christ, that with quietness they work, and eat their own bread. (II Thessalonians 3:10-12)

Explanation of connection
There are several things that God says are like spiritual food to us. These are chiefly God Himself, the written Word of God, fellowship with other Christians, and our work. A loss of appetite therefore indicates that we have lost our spiritual appetite for these things.

God has also instructed man that he must work in order to eat (Genesis 3:19), so when we cease to work, we may lose our appetite. This attitude may in turn come from a slow metabolism (see *Thyroid, page 174)*.

Way of healing
Confess your lack of appetite for God, for the Bible, fellowship, or for work.

Helpful scriptures
Matthew 6:33; Ecclesiastes 5:19

Endocrine

Spiritual meaning: **instincts**

Scriptures
- For that which I do I allow not: for what I would, that do I not; but what I hate, that do I. If then I do that which I would not, I consent unto the law that it is good. Now then it is no more I that do it, but sin that dwelleth in me. For I know that in me (that is, in my flesh,) dwelleth no good thing: for to will is present with me; but how to perform that which is good I find not. For the good that I would I do not: but the evil which I would not, that I do. Now if I do that I would not, it is no more I that do it, but sin that dwelleth in me (Romans 7:13-20)

Explanation of connection
A hormone is a chemical substance which is produced in one part of the body and is carried in the blood stream to another part of the body where it causes certain things to happen. It is a kind of instant biological message. An example is adrenalin which is released in response to certain mental sensations such as fear or excitement, and prepares the body for sudden action by (amongst other things) increasing blood-sugar levels, increasing heart rate and dilating the pupils of the eyes.

Hormones are therefore instinctive responses working secondary to the functions of the brain. The brain makes certain decisions and judgements, and the hormones automatically work in response to these. A message carried by hormones obviously differs from a neurological signal (carried by nerves directly from the brain).

In spiritual terms, therefore, hormones speak of our automatic response to things. For example, it is instinctive for a woman to be motherly. If this instinct is too strong, it will be indicated by an increase in the hormone and size of the relevant gland; if the instinct is weak, the hormone and gland will be reduced. If the instinct is simply wrong and tainted by sin, the gland may become diseased. Whether our instincts work as they should is decided by the current condition of our minds. The natural unsaved man has a carnal, sinful mind. This means that his automatic response to circumstances is sinful.

> The carnal mind is enmity against God: for it is not subject to the law of God, neither indeed can be. So then they that are in the flesh cannot please God. (Romans 8:7-8)
> They are of the world: therefore speak they of the world, and the world heareth them. (I John 4:5)

The man who is born again and is walking in the Spirit, has a new mind, which pleases God, and his automatic response is Godly.

> And hereby we do know that we know him, if we keep his commandments. He that saith, I know him, and keepeth not his commandments, is a liar, and the truth is not in him. (I John 2:3-4)
> We know that we have passed from death unto life, because we love the brethren. He that loveth not his brother abideth in death. (I John 3:14)
> The fruit of the Spirit is love, joy, peace, longsuffering, gentleness, goodness, faith, Meekness, temperance: against such there is no law. (Galations 5:22-23).

If we have the mind of Christ, we will automatically do the things that please Him, but if our mind is carnal, we will automatically sin. All sins that we commit are the result of having a carnal mind. If we allow our mind to be fleshly, we will not be able to stop ourselves sinning.

In order to have the mind of Christ, to be walking in the Spirit, it is necessary to spend time with the Lord. That is why it is important to begin each day with communion with Him, reading the Bible and praying, so that He gives us His Spirit. Then, if we have truly met with Him, through the day we will naturally be in the Spirit and therefore producing the fruit of the Spirit.

Physical hormonal problems indicate fleshly responses due to a fleshly mind.

Adrenaline is the body's response to fear or excitement, stimulating the whole body ready for action. This speaks of a person's spiritual excitement. Obviously, it is necessary to keep the balance between overexcitement and unresponsiveness. Genuine spiritual stirring in response to things of the Holy Spirit is right and proper, but excitement over fleshy ideas needs to be avoided. A person with the mind of Christ will be able to discern between the two, and therefore respond appropriately.

Testosterone speaks of essentially male characteristics. These include strength and authority which a man exercises in loving, protecting and ruling his household *(for references see also page 135)*. If a man submits to women, fails to wisely govern his household or area of responsibility, fails to protect, he is failing to fulfil his role as a man. Excess testosterone will indicate a man who is too strong in these spheres, and insufficient testosterone, a man who is too weak. (Women also have testosterone, inasmuch as women in part need to adopt male characteristics of authority etc., such as when dealing with children. An excess will indicate too much dominance, too little will indicate weakness).

Oestrogens speak of essentially female characteristics *(for references see page 135)*. A woman's normal role is to nourish and bring up children, to care and look after people, to assist her husband and be in subjection to him. This indicates gentleness and care. A person with excess oestrogens will be too gentle; with insufficient they will be not gentle and caring enough.

Growth Hormone

This speaks of spiritual growth, of growing to maturity. A person who is big in their own eyes, will in fact be very small; those that think they are mature, will in fact be very immature. A lack of growth hormone indicates a person who is great in their own eyes and so is small. Excess growth hormone indicates a person who is small in their own eyes.

We see this in the case of Saul, who, though he was head and shoulders above his peers in height, he thought of himself as very small, hiding amongst the baggage (I Samuel 10:22-23). Later, after his character changed, Samuel says of him:

> When thou wast little in thine own sight, wast thou not made the head of the tribes of Israel, and the LORD anointed thee king over Israel? (I Samuel 15:17)

The purpose of this is remedial. When someone is very big in their own eyes, God may make them small physically in order to humble them, and vice versa. Unfortunately, as with Saul, people can then go too far the other way.

Being small in one's own eyes also causes the individual to strive to do more – to grow, to improve oneself, to be more useful, rather than being restful and content. This will be evident in cases of acromegaly, when the sufferer feels they have never done enough for their family *(see* Bones).

Way of healing
Confess that a particular instinct is wrong. Confess also that your instincts are wrong in general because you don't have the mind of Christ. Confess that you have not been going to the Lord and receiving His mind. Spend time with Him, turning from the things of the world and giving yourself totally to Him as a living sacrifice, so that He may transform your mind and bring your healing.

Helpful scriptures
Romans 12:1-2

Thyroid

Spiritual meaning: relates to faith/zeal

Scriptures
- Above all, taking the shield of faith, wherewith ye shall be able to quench all the fiery darts of the wicked. (Ephesians 6:16)
- Having then gifts differing according to the grace that is given to us, whether prophecy, let us prophesy according to the proportion of faith. (Romans 12:6)
- For unto us was the gospel preached, as well as unto them: but the word preached did not profit them, not being mixed with faith in them that heard it. (Hebrews 4:2)
- Then touched he their eyes, saying, According to your faith be it unto you. (Matthew 9:29)

Explanation of connection

The thyroid gland produces hormones which regulate the rate at which different parts of the body operate and grow. An overactive thyroid gland makes the body's systems work too quickly, leaving a person feeling agitated, restless and hot. An under-active thyroid gland makes the body's systems work too slowly, leaving a person feeling lethargic, listless and cold. A malfunctioning thyroid gland has far-reaching effects on the whole of the body.

The spiritual equivalent is *faith*. Faith regulates the speed at which we live our spiritual lives. Someone with much faith will be living the Christian life with much energy, enthusiasm and at a great pace; a person with little faith will have little interest or involvement in spiritual things, moving at a very slow pace. A lack of faith, therefore, has far-reaching effects over the whole of the spiritual life.

The word *thyroid* comes from the Greek for 'like a shield', because the gland, and the cartilage above it (the Adam's apple), are both shaped like an oblong Greek shield. The connection is evident in Ephesians 6, where Paul says,

> Above all, taking the shield [Greek: *thureos*] of faith, wherewith ye shall be able to quench all the fiery darts of the wicked. (Ephesians 6:16)

A person who is full of faith and Godly enthusiasm is able to quench any attack the enemy throws at him.

To have faith means in practice to believe God, to trust Him and take Him at His word. In Hebrews 11 it speaks extensively on the subject of faith, saying that the men of faith in the Old Testament did not live according to what they could see, but according to what God had promised.

> Now faith is the substance of things hoped for, the evidence of things not seen. ...By faith Abraham, when he was called to go out into a place which he should after receive for an

inheritance, obeyed; and he went out, not knowing whither he went. ...For he looked for a city which hath foundations, whose builder and maker is God. (Hebrews 11:1, 8, 10)

When the disciples said to the Lord Jesus, increase our faith, He replied:

If ye had faith as a grain of mustard seed, ye might say unto this sycamine tree, Be thou plucked up by the root, and be thou planted in the sea; and it should obey you. (Luke 17:5)

The Lord was saying that you don't need to *receive* faith, but if you exercise faith, if you truly believe God in just the smallest way, you will start to see great things happen.

A person with hypothyroidism will be lacking in faith. A person with hyperthyroidism will have too much zeal.

Too much zeal

There are times when we believe so strongly that God can do anything, that we get carried away with zeal and excited enthusiasm. We can start to move out and act without being instructed by the Lord, and consequently can make serious mistakes. We see examples of this amongst the apostles, such as Peter when he said,

Though I should die with thee, yet will I not deny thee. (Matthew 26:35).

Similarly, Thomas said,

Let us also go, that we may die with him. (John 11:16)

Though the disciples had the right attitude, they were rushing ahead. Too much enthusiastic zeal is counter-productive, so it is important to learn to wait upon the Lord, to be guided by Him and to go at the pace He sets.

Way of healing

a. Hypothyroidism

Confess that you haven't been keeping your eyes on eternal matters and values, that you have been living according to what you can see. See that this world is temporary and that the things of God are eternal. See the necessity of believing what God has said and of living your life accordingly. Then ask for your healing.

Helpful scriptures

Hebrews 11:1-12:3;

b. Hyperthyroidism

Confess that you have become carried away with zeal, and been restless rather than resting in God. Remember that He says that *He* will build His church (Matthew 16:18) and that we only have to move at His command, never before.

Eyes

Spiritual meaning: **spiritual vision**

Scriptures

- The LORD is in his holy temple, the LORD's throne is in heaven: his eyes behold, his eyelids try, the children of men. (Psalm 11:4)
- Son of man, thou dwellest in the midst of a rebellious house, which have eyes to see, and see not; they have ears to hear, and hear not: for they are a rebellious house. (Ezekiel 12:2)
- And why beholdest thou the mote that is in thy brother's eye, but considerest not the beam that is in thine own eye? Or how wilt thou say to thy brother, Let me pull out the mote out of thine eye; and, behold, a beam is in thine own eye? Thou hypocrite, first cast out the beam out of thine own eye; and then shalt thou see clearly to cast out the mote out of thy brother's eye. (Matthew 7:3-5)

Explanation of connection

Our physical sight symbolises our spiritual sight, our spiritual discernment. Thus, in the verses quoted above, it speaks of the Lord's eyes discerning mankind's heart. Similarly, in Matthew 7, a person with sin in their heart will not have the spiritual discernment to deal with someone else's sin.

Any loss of sight therefore indicates a loss of spiritual discernment and vision. It means we have failed to see things as they really are. There may be various reasons for this. Sin of any kind in our lives hinders our vision. John says,

> But he that hateth his brother is in darkness, and walketh in darkness, and knoweth not whither he goeth, because that darkness hath blinded his eyes. (I John 2:11)

As long as we allow sins to remain in our lives and are unwilling to confess them and turn from them, then we are walking in darkness, even as Christians.

Yet any failure to see things as they really are may bring impaired eyesight.

a) Focussing on appearances, lusting with the eyes,

- Thou shalt not wrest judgment; thou shalt not respect persons, neither take a gift: for a gift doth blind the eyes of the wise, and pervert the words of the righteous. (Deuteronomy 16:19)
- He that hasteth to be rich hath an evil eye, and considereth not that poverty shall come upon him. (Proverbs 28:22)
- When goods increase, they are increased that eat them: and what good is there to the owners thereof, saving the beholding of them with their eyes? (Ecclesiastes: 5:11)
- Better is the sight of the eyes than the wandering of the desire: this is also vanity and vexation of spirit. (Ecclesiastes: 6:9)

If we focus on appearances, it means we are not seeing things as they really are: we are looking at the outward, not at the spiritual reality. Because our spiritual eyesight is impaired, our physical eyesight may follow suit.

It is very easy for us to misuse our eyes, by using them to lust after things. When we see something beautiful, we start to desire it, to want it for ourselves. It may be a material possession – a new car or house – or it may be a person that we lust after. We may be very taken up with the appearance of things: how we look, how other people look, the appearance of our houses. All of these are examples of 'the lust of the eyes' (I John 2:16).

One of the things that attracted Eve to the forbidden fruit in Genesis 3 was its appearance.

> And when the woman saw that the tree was… pleasant to the eyes she took of the fruit thereof, and did eat, and gave also unto her husband with her; and he did eat. (Genesis 3:6)

As Christians, we are to be spiritual people, considering things from God's point of view rather than being interested in physical appearances.

When God sent Samuel to anoint a King to replace Saul, He sent Him to the household of Jesse. When the eldest son is brought before Samuel, the Lord reveals to Samuel how he is to view him.

> But the LORD said unto Samuel, Look not on his countenance, or on the height of his stature; because I have refused him: for the LORD seeth not as man seeth; for man looketh on the outward appearance, but the LORD looketh on the heart. (I Samuel 16:7)

We are told not to be 'respecters of persons' (James 2:1-5). That means, we are not to be influenced by the way people dress, how they look, how rich they are, who they are: we are to view them spiritually as God does.

Equally, when we have to buy something we need, like a new house or car, we must be careful not to lust after the appearance: we must get what is practical and what God wants us to have, rather than what our eyes desire.

In our own appearance, it is to be expected that we should make ourselves look pleasant, but we can do this without too much thought, time and effort, without becoming obsessed.

How healing comes

Confess to the Lord that you have been focusing on appearances. You have cared about how things look; you have lusted with your eyes. Realise that spiritual things are what really matter: our interest in people should be in how they are spiritually, not how they look physically; our possessions should be there as tools to serve God and should never become our focus.

Helpful scriptures

Colossians 3:1-11

b) Grief

Scriptures:

- And the man of thine, whom I shall not cut off from mine altar, shall be to consume thine eyes, and to grieve thine heart: and all the increase of thine house shall die in the flower of their age. (1 Samuel 2:33)
- Have mercy upon me, O LORD, for I am in trouble: mine eye is consumed with grief, yea, my soul and my belly. (Psalm 31:9) [The word *grief* comes from a root meaning *to be angry, be grieved, take indignation, provoke (to anger, unto wrath), have sorrow, vex, be wroth.*]

When we are grieving over something, or harbouring a grievance, it may become such a focus of our lives that we fail to see things as they really are - we lose our spiritual sight. As we gaze on something we love and are grieved by what we see, it is like something eating away at our eyes.

When Eli the priest was an old man, he allowed his sons to behave wickedly: they stole the best of the sacrificial meat for themselves and lay with women at the door of the tabernacle. Eli looked on and was grieved, pleading with them to stop. However, he didn't actually force them to stop as he should have done. God held him responsible for not taking proper steps against his sons:

> Wherefore… honourest thy sons above me, to make yourselves fat with the chiefest of all the offerings of Israel my people? (I Samuel 2:29)

God says that one of the consequences will be that his eyes will be eaten away because of his children:

> And the man of thine, whom I shall not cut off from mine altar, shall be to consume thine eyes, and to grieve thine heart: and all the increase of thine house shall die in the flower of their age. And this shall be a sign unto thee, that shall come upon thy two sons, on Hophni and Phinehas; in one day they shall die both of them. (I Samuel 2:33, 34)

Eli's problem was that he looked at his sons and loved them for what they appeared to be, no doubt fine looking young men, rather than what he knew them to be – wicked men who were defiling the sanctuary. He has made idols of his sons. As he looks on these idols, his heart is grieved because they are behaving so abominably. Yet he does nothing about it. Consequently, he is responsible for his own grief. He continues to gaze on his wayward sons and does nothing about them until his eyes grow dim.

> Eli was laid down in his place, and his eyes began to wax dim, that he could not see. (1 Samuel 3:2)

His wrong attitude towards his children clouded his spiritual vision and his physical vision was also affected.

Our eyes may be filled with grief because we have lost something we longed after: perhaps we wanted a possession, perhaps an inheritance, and it went to another. We have been grieving over it: looking at it with our mind's eye, but being eaten up by the fact that it has been taken from us. This could be true of a loved one we have lost or a chance we have missed. We start to put the thing before God, gazing at it and being consumed with grief.

How healing comes

God says that He alone is to be our God, the one whom we serve.

> Thou shalt have no other gods before me. Thou shalt not make unto thee any graven image, or any likeness of any thing that is in heaven above, or that is in the earth beneath, or that is in the water under the earth. Thou shalt not bow down thyself to them, nor serve them. (Exodus 20:3-5)

When we have lost something, even when we have lost a loved one, if we spend our time focusing on that person or thing, and being grieved by our loss, we are committing idolatry. It is worshipping the person, the thing. Consequently our spiritual vision is affected. God requires us to find our all in all in Him, and in Him alone: to be taken up with Him and to serve Him. He is the one in whom we are to find our happiness and the satisfaction of our hearts.

Confess that you have been grieving over something: trust in the Lord, let Him be your God and take your eyes off the subject of your grief.

Your spiritual eyesight will return and you may ask for your physical healing.

Short-sightedness

Some people can only see their immediate situation, not the big picture. They think only about day to day affairs, about the things immediately concerning themselves. They lose sight of how God is working things out in the long-term, and the fact that God works on a vast scale. They may become worried because they can only see a short distance. This is the cause of short-sightedness.

How healing comes

Remember that God works to a long term plan. After all, it was about four thousand years into the history of the world that Christ came.

Confess that you have been taken up with your current situation, rather than seeing the wider scheme of things. God will work things out for His glory and our good, whatever the current circumstances. He says,

> For I know the thoughts that I think toward you, saith the LORD, thoughts of peace, and not of evil, to give you an expected end. (Jeremiah 29:11)

Helpful scriptures
II Kings 6:1-17

Long-sightedness

Some people think so much about the big picture that they cannot focus on what they are supposed to be doing at the moment, the work in hand. They may think all about the future and where their life may be leading, about God's great purposes in history and across the world and the wider church, and lose sight of the immediate situation and the job God has given them for today.

The way of healing

Confess that you haven't kept your mind on the job in hand, that your focus has become too distant, too broad. God says,

> Seek ye first the kingdom of God, and his righteousness; and all these things shall be added unto you. Take therefore no thought for the morrow: for the morrow shall take thought for the things of itself. Sufficient unto the day is the evil thereof. (Matthew 6:34)

Balance

Having read the causes of short- and long-sightedness, you may think that they are contradictory. The point is that our sight of the big picture should never become so out of hand that we cannot focus on the immediate and vice versa. We should hold the two in balance.

Squint (strabismus)

A squint is when the eyes do not look in the same direction. This speaks of a person who is not single-minded, especially for the things of God. They may have various things in their lives that distract them and stop them focusing on Christ and His kingdom. The Lord Jesus speaks of being 'single-eyed':

> The light of the body is the eye: therefore when thine eye is single, thy whole body also is full of light; but when thine eye is evil, thy body also is full of darkness. (Luke 11:34)

He goes on to explain that being single-eyed means having the whole of one's being devoted to God, and having no dark, hidden part.

> If thy whole body therefore be full of light, having no part dark, the whole shall be full of light, as when the bright shining of a candle doth give thee light. (Luke 11:36)

Way of healing

See that you need to be single-minded for the things of God, focusing on Him. He promises that if we seek first His kingdom, He will take care of everything else.

> Seek ye first the kingdom of God, and his righteousness; and all these things shall be added unto you. (Matthew 6:33)

Confess that you have allowed other things to come into your life so you are not fully focused on serving God and living for Him.

Helpful Scriptures

Matthew 6:19-34; I John 1;

Fatigue, including chronic fatigue syndrome and ME, insomnia (*see also* Digestive System *for related symptoms*)

Spiritual cause: **Lack of rest**

Scriptures:
- Six years thou shalt sow thy field, and six years thou shalt prune thy vineyard, and gather in the fruit thereof; but in the seventh year shall be a sabbath of rest unto the land, a sabbath for the LORD: thou shalt neither sow thy field, nor prune thy vineyard. That which groweth of its own accord of thy harvest thou shalt not reap, neither gather the grapes of thy vine undressed: for it is a year of rest unto the land. (Leviticus 25:3-5)
- And if ye will not for all this hearken unto me, but walk contrary unto me; then I will walk contrary unto you also in fury; and I, even I, will chastise you seven times for your sins. Then shall the land enjoy her sabbaths, as long as it lieth desolate, and ye be in your enemies' land; even then shall the land rest, and enjoy her sabbaths. As long as it lieth desolate it shall rest; because it did not rest in your sabbaths, when ye dwelt upon it. (Leviticus 26:27-28; 34-35)

Explanation of connection
There is a principle in Scripture that when something does not get its true rest, rest is forced upon it. In the scriptures quoted above, God decrees that even the land should receive its due rest. Every seventh year, the land is to lie fallow – neither sown nor harvested – simply left alone to renew itself ready for the next six years.

The Lord says that if His people disobey Him, then He will ensure that the land receives its rest – by removing the people from the land so that the land lies desolate.

We see in history that this is exactly what happens. In II Chronicles 36:20-21, it says that Judah was taken into captivity so that the land should enjoy her sabbaths – her due rest.

And them that had escaped from the sword carried he away to Babylon; where they were servants to him and his sons until the reign of the kingdom of Persia: to fulfil the word of the LORD by the mouth of Jeremiah, until the land had enjoyed her sabbaths: for as long as she lay desolate she kept sabbath, to fulfil threescore and ten years. (II Chronicles 36:20-21)

God has also ordained rest for humans. He says

Remember the sabbath day, to keep it holy. Six days shalt thou labour, and do all thy work: but the seventh day is the sabbath of the LORD thy God: in it thou shalt not do any work, thou, nor thy son, nor thy daughter, thy manservant, nor thy maidservant, nor thy cattle, nor thy stranger that is within thy gates: for in six days the LORD made heaven and earth, the sea, and all that in them is, and rested the seventh day: wherefore the LORD blessed the sabbath day, and hallowed it. (Exodus 20:8-11)

Many people have complicated the idea of a sabbath, but biblically it is fairly simple. We need one day a week when we stop working altogether and simply rest.[26] That means no housework, no catching up with paid work: simply rest. Rest really means quietness and taking a break from activity. This may involve various forms of true relaxation, but no kind of work. We should also take, from time to time, longer holidays. God ordained certain feasts in the calendar of Israel, so we should equally take time during the year for holidays. We should also allow ourselves to rest in the evenings after our day's work: God gave us the darkness so that we should learn to work in the day and rest at night, that is, when it gets dark. This truth comes out when Jesus says:

I must work the works of him who sent me, while it is day. The night is coming, when no one can work. (John 9:4)

It is also important to find time for a true rest in the middle of a working day. This will bring increased efficiency. (Note, however,

---

[26] The day on which we rest does not matter. Paul says, 'One man esteemeth one day above another: another esteemeth every day alike. Let every man be fully persuaded in his own mind' (Romans 14:5).

that we are told to work six days. A lack of proper work on six days will make it hard to rest on the seventh).

Some people find it very difficult to rest. They have to be doing something continually; they can't sit still. They are bored if they have to relax. They will typically do several things at once: eat lunch, read a book, listen to the radio, and may even get up in the middle of all this to put some washing on. When they go on holiday, they take work with them.

Therefore, when people do not take the rest ordained for them, they suffer from fatigue, which forces them to rest.

There is, however, a deeper reason for the inability to rest: a lack of spiritual rest. As Christians, the New Testament says, we have been provided with a spiritual rest:

> There remaineth therefore a rest to the people of God. For he that is entered into his rest, he also hath ceased from his own works, as God did from his. (Hebrews 4:9, 10)

When we became Christians, we discovered that we did not have to work to receive our salvation: the Lord Jesus, in dying on the cross for us, achieved this: He did the work for us. There is nothing left to pay – we can rest in our salvation because Christ has finished the work.

What is more, now we are saved, the work that we have to do in living the Christian life is still Christ's to perform: all we have to do is to trust Him and obey, and leave Him to do the work. In that we have ceased from working (doing the work ourselves), we can enter into our rest.

> Wherefore, my beloved, as ye have always obeyed, not as in my presence only, but now much more in my absence, work out your own salvation with fear and trembling. For **it is God which worketh in you both to will and to do of his good pleasure**. (Philippians 2:12, 13)

Since we can trust Christ to perfect the work He has begun in us (Philippians 1:6), and trust Him to look after us and never leave us (Hebrews 13:5), we can be in a perpetual state of spiritual rest, even when we are working. We can relax, knowing that God is sovereign.

When we feel that we are responsible for everything and don't have spiritual rest, it causes us to keep working and never relax. We quickly become fatigued. The person who feels that it is up to him to maintain his own salvation will lack spiritual rest.

Rest in Christ

We may also have feelings of discontentment. The Bible says that everything we need is in Christ.

> Blessed be the God and Father of our Lord Jesus Christ, who hath blessed us with all spiritual blessings in heavenly places in Christ. (Ephesians 1:3)

If we are not finding everything we need in Christ, if we are always seeking after joy, fulfilment, pleasure and rest in other things (such as service), we will not have spiritual rest. It will cause us to be always on the move, always working, never sitting still. We may be always thinking about what is going to happen in the future, rather than finding Christ to be our sufficiency in the present. Augustine said of God,

> Thou hast made us for thyself, and our hearts are restless till they find their rest in Thee.[27]

Christ calls us to come to Him and find Him to be our all in all so that our hearts might be at rest.

Insomnia

Another symptom of lacking spiritual rest is insomnia, so all that has been written above applies here as well. The person who has truly found his rest in Christ will be able to sleep soundly.

Food, digestion and fatigue

Fatigue can also be due to an inadequate diet, food intolerance, or a problem assimilating nutrients. *See* <u>Digestive system</u>, *page 146.*

---

[27] Augustine of Hippo, *Confessions* I.i.1

How healing comes

Admit that you haven't come to find your rest in Christ, that you are trying to live your Christian life in your own strength. Perhaps you feel discontent and are consequently always on the move. You don't take time to rest and relax.

See that Christ Himself is all that you need, the only one who can satisfy your heart: rest in Him, and He will heal your fatigue.

Helpful scriptures

Proverbs 3:5; Hebrews 13:5-6; I Corinthians 7:18-31

Feet and legs (*see also* <u>Hip</u>, <u>Knee</u>)

Spiritual meaning

- **Where confidence is placed**
- **Associations**
- **The spiritual walk**

Scriptures – see below

Explanation of connection

In the physical realm, our feet have two main functions. They are the part of the body on which we stand and they are the means by which we walk.

In spiritual terms, the feet speak to us of where we place our confidence and the way in which we conduct our spiritual walk.

Confidence

Psalm 40 says,

> He brought me up also out of an horrible pit, out of the miry clay, and set my feet upon a rock, and established my goings. (Psalm 40:2)

Our confidence in all things should be in God. He is the firm, unshakable Rock on whom we stand. If we place our trust in something else, it is like trying to stand on diseased feet.

> Confidence in an unfaithful man in time of trouble is like a
> broken tooth, and a foot out of joint. (Proverbs 25:19)

A notable figure in the Old Testament who put his trust in man
and not in God was King Asa of Judah. When his enemy the
King of Israel is making preparations to beseige Judah, Asa takes
silver and gold out of the treasures of the Lord's house and sends
them to the King of Syria, asking him to come to his aid. The
King of Syria duly obliges. In response to this, however, the Lord
rebukes Asa:

> And at that time Hanani the seer came to Asa king of Judah,
> and said unto him, Because thou hast relied on the king of
> Syria, and not relied on the LORD thy God, therefore is the host
> of the king of Syria escaped out of thine hand. (II Chronicles
> 16:7)

As well as the rebuke, King Asa receives a disease:

> And Asa in the thirty and ninth year of his reign was diseased
> in his feet, until his disease was exceeding great. (II Chronicles
> 16:12)

Asa had been trusting in man rather than in God, so the disease
he receives is in his feet. What is interesting, however, is his
response to the disease:

> Yet in his disease he sought not to the LORD, but to the
> physicians. (II Chronicles 16:12)

In his disease, he repeats his mistake by trusting in the physicians
to heal him rather than God.

Similarly, it is clear in the case of the lame man by the pool of
Bethesda that he had been trusting in man to help him. He says,

> I have no man, when the water is troubled, to put me into the
> pool: but while I am coming, another steppeth down before
> me. (John 5:7)

Diseased feet may therefore indicate that we put our confidence in men rather than in God.

Associations

King Asa had a league with the King of Syria, and as a result of this, when times were difficult, he turned to him for help. However, it was wrong of him to have an association with an enemy of God, with someone whom he should have been overthrowing. It says in Amos,

> Can two walk together, except they be agreed? (Amos 3:3)

We may have alliances in our lives which are inappropriate for us as Christians. We may have certain associations with things that are ungodly. It may be the television, the pub, ungodly friends. We don't really trust in them in times of ease – we just associate with them. But when times are difficult, we may be quickly led to fall back onto them, to try to find our help and reassurance in them. It makes it clear in Proverbs that we should not walk with these people, should not associate with them, because they will lead us to sin.

> My son, walk not thou in the way with them; refrain thy foot from their path: for their feet run to evil, and make haste to shed blood. (Proverbs 1:15, 16)

We may find that if we have worldly associations that we suffer problems with our feet. Small associations may bring minor difficulties, increasing to severe problems with major associations.

A strong spiritual walk

Another important fact with regard to our feet and legs is having a strong spiritual walk. We are told that Enoch walked with God (Genesis 5:24), as did Noah (Genesis 6:9). That means that they spent time with Him, and grew in grace and in knowledge of Him; they moved forward.

As believers, we need to have a positive on-going walk with God. Perhaps we are being weak in our walk and remaining where we are spiritually, rather than moving forward. Perhaps God has told us to take the next step, perhaps through baptism or active Christian service and we have not taken it. (This will also depend upon having your trust firmly in God, as has already been discussed – the walk is dependent upon the feet.) An inability to walk physically will indicate that we have become unable to walk spiritually.

There are various things that will stop us moving forward spiritually. Sins may be left undealt with; we may have become resigned to our current spiritual state and stopped seeking an ever deeper experience of God.

It is interesting to read in Acts of two men who couldn't walk, both of whom were suffering from weakness in their feet. These are both unsaved men, but when they trust in Christ and their spiritual walk begins, they receive strength in their feet.

> And there sat a certain man at Lystra, impotent in his feet, being a cripple from his mother's womb, who never had walked: the same heard Paul speak: who stedfastly beholding him, and perceiving that he had faith to be healed, said with a loud voice, Stand upright on thy feet. And he leaped and walked. (Acts 14:8-10 – *see also* Acts 3:1-8)

Our walk also speaks of our service for God. Isaiah speaks of the beauty of feet that serve the Lord in spreading the gospel.

> How beautiful upon the mountains are the feet of him that bringeth good tidings, that publisheth peace; that bringeth good tidings of good, that publisheth salvation; that saith unto Zion, Thy God reigneth! (Isaiah 52:7)

For this reason, it says in Ephesians that we should have our 'feet shod with the preparation of the gospel of peace' (Ephesians

6:15). The weakness in our spiritual walk may thus relate to service.

Regain your strength by waiting upon God to enable you to move forward with Him.

Hallux valgus

Perhaps surprisingly, Scripture does speak about big toes (see Leviticus 14:14 and 8:23). Since the big toe leads the rest of the foot, it speaks of our leadership in the field of our associations, friendships. A *hallux valgus,* therefore, which is when the big toe is bent towards the other toes and often squashes them, indicates an overly-interested and domineering attitude towards associates.

Nails – *see under* Hand and Arm, *page 197.*

Unequal legs

- The legs of the lame are not equal: so is a parable in the mouth of fools. (Proverbs 26:6, 7)

Unequal legs are a sign of an inequality in the spiritual walk. Part of the person's life is lived in accordance with the will of God, but part is not. You may be seeking to live a Christian life without being wholly committed to God.

How healing comes

See that it's necessary to have a walk with God, in which your trust is fully in Him. Confess that you have associated with things that are worldly and ungodly and have perhaps been going to the world and to man for help, rather than going to God. Confess that your walk with God has become slack.

Helpful Scriptures

Proverbs 3:5-8

Legs

- He delighteth not in the strength of the horse: he taketh not pleasure in the legs of a man. (Psalm 147:10)
- His legs are as pillars of marble, set upon sockets of fine gold: his countenance is as Lebanon, excellent as the cedars. (Song of Solomon 5:15)

The *leg* properly refers to a combination of the hip, thigh, knee, shin and ankle, which should be seen individually. As a combination they stand for a person's strength in standing and moving spiritually.

Shin

- And he had greaves of brass upon his legs. (I Samuel 17:6)
- Wherefore let him that thinketh he standeth take heed lest he fall. (I Corinthians 10:12)

The Hebrew word for *greaves* (shin-armour) comes from a word meaning 'conspicuous'. The shin is the conspicuous thing which keeps us upright, which shows that we are standing. When our shin is damaged, it means that we are no longer standing spiritually but have taken a fall. This comes about when we try to stand in our own strength, rather than in the Lord's: when we think we can stand, we are likely to fall.

Helpful Scriptures
Proverbs 3:5, 6

Haemorrhoids

Spiritual cause: **losing sight of grace**

Scriptures
- When the Philistines took the ark of God, they brought it into the house of Dagon, and set it by Dagon. But the hand of the LORD was heavy upon them of Ashdod, and he destroyed

them, and smote them with emerods, even Ashdod and
the coasts thereof. (I Samuel 5:6)

- And it was so, that, after they had carried it about, the
  hand of the LORD was against the city with a very great
  destruction: and he smote the men of the city, both small
  and great, and they had emerods in their secret parts. (I
  Samuel 5:9)

Explanation of connection

Haemorrhoids are swollen veins either internal or external to
the anal sphincter. The veins become inflamed and often bleed.
Haemorrhoids may be caused by an increase in pressure on the
region, such as through pregnancy or lifting a heavy object,
or through straining as a result of constipation, or by a local
infection.

In spiritual terms, they indicate a loss of spiritual life through
putting too much pressure on ourselves and other people, often
through trying too hard. We may summarise this as losing sight
of grace.

Haemorrhoids in Scripture

When the Philistines stole the Ark of the Covenant and brought
it to Ashdod, they hid it in the house of their god Dagon. Then,
we are told, they were smitten with haemorrhoids.

But the hand of the LORD was heavy upon them of Ashdod,
and he destroyed them, and smote them with emerods, even
Ashdod and the coasts thereof. (I Samuel 5:6)

The same thing happened in Gath and Ekron when the Ark was
moved there.

In the Old Testament, the Ark of the Covenant, including the
Mercy Seat, was the place on which the sacrificial blood was
poured out each year on the Day of Atonement. Having stolen
this and hidden it in a secret place, the disease that the Philistines
get is described thus:

Emerods [bleeding veins] in their secret parts (I Samuel 5:9)

The bleeding veins in a hidden part of their body represented the fact that they had hidden the Mercy Seat where blood was placed. Inasmuch as the Ark represented the mercy and grace of God, when we get haemorrhoids it is an indication that we have hidden God's grace, or lost sight of it.

Grace is the showing of unmerited favour. As Christians we receive this from God, his goodness and kindness to us which does not depend upon who we are and what we deserve. Our salvation and forgiveness comes to us entirely as a gift from God, which we receive by confession of sin and faith, not by works.

> ...Being justified freely by his grace through the redemption that is in Christ Jesus. (Romans 3:24)

Just as our salvation was a gift of grace, so our lives as Christians are to be lived by grace: we should simply be trusting in the goodness of God to guide our lives, and not live them in our own strength. Every good thing that happens occurs entirely by the grace and goodness of God, not because of us.

> ...Being confident of this very thing, that he which hath begun a good work in you will perform it until the day of Jesus Christ. (Philippians 1:6)

However, sometimes we lose sight of God's grace, and think that everything depends upon us. We become legalistic, and try and earn God's favour by our actions. We strive to do more and more by way of Christian service to try and win His favour. We have an unmerciful attitude towards ourselves. We fail to see that God's forgiveness is freely available to all who come to Him admitting their failure.

A lack of realisation of God's grace causes us to show a lack of grace towards others. We may make our favour and kindness dependent upon their actions, rather than letting it be unconditional. We may show a lack of forgiveness. We may be a hard taskmaster and show a lack of mercy.

There is a strong link between a lack of grace and a lack of mercy. Consequently, people with haemorrhoids very often also have <u>constipation</u>.

Way of healing
Confess that you have lost sight of God's grace for yourself and other people. You have failed to see that His favour and His forgiveness come not as a result of our getting everything right, but simply as a free gift when we admit our failure, our sinfulness and our need. See that it is necessary to demonstrate the grace of God towards other people, forgiving them when they harm us. Then ask for your healing.

Helpful scriptures
Ephesians 2:4-17; James 1:17

Hand and Arm

Spiritual meaning: relates to work/actions

Scriptures
- Whatsoever thy hand findeth to do, do it with thy might. (Ecclesiastes 9:10)
- He becometh poor that dealeth with a slack hand: but the hand of the diligent maketh rich. He that gathereth in summer is a wise son: but he that sleepeth in harvest is a son that causeth shame. (Proverbs 10:4-5)

Explanation of connection
Inasmuch as our hands are the agents by which we do our work, when there is something amiss in the realm of our service, our hands become injured or diseased. This may include:
- failing to do those things that we should
- using our hands for things we shouldn't do (because it keeps us from our real work)
- having a bad attitude towards our fellow-workers.

Stretching out our hands for good

One of the key things that we are to do as Christians is to stretch out our hands to help other people. This is described in Proverbs 31 as one of the marks of a Godly woman:

> She stretcheth out her hand to the poor; yea, she reacheth forth her hands to the needy. (Proverbs 31:1)

When we are unwilling to stretch out our hands to help others, we may find that our physical hand ceases to function, perhaps being unable to stretch out.

The Lord Jesus spoke about this in a remarkable incident. On a particular occasion, when He had gone into a synagogue on the sabbath day, there was a man there with an infirmity. It says that those that were there asked Him,

> Is it lawful to heal on the sabbath days? that they might accuse him. And he said unto them, What man shall there be among you, that shall have one sheep, and if it fall into a pit on the sabbath day, will he not lay hold on it, and lift it out? How much then is a man better than a sheep? Wherefore it is lawful to do well on the sabbath days. (Matthew 12:10-12)

The Lord Jesus is clearly teaching them that, when it lies in their power to help someone, they should stretch out their hand to do so.

> Withhold not good from them to whom it is due, when it is in the power of thine hand to do it. (Proverbs 3:27)

But what was the illness that the man was suffering from? A withered hand.

> Then saith he to the man, Stretch forth thine hand. And he stretched it forth; and it was restored whole, like as the other. (Matthew 12:13)

It seems that the Lord's explanation is for the sake of the ill man. No doubt he has suffered the withered hand as a result of not stretching out his hand himself, of not reaching out to help others, to care for the poor and needy. The Lord therefore teaches him the importance of this in preparation for his healing.

Though man is often unwilling to stretch out his hands for others, God is never like this. Isaiah says,

> Behold, the LORD's hand is not shortened, that it cannot save. (Isaiah 59:1)

Moreover, the Lord Jesus, when he went to the cross stretched out both his hands in order to save us. In Psalm 88, a messianic Psalm speaking of the Lord Jesus on the cross it says,

> Mine eye mourneth by reason of affliction: LORD, I have called daily upon thee, I have stretched out my hands unto thee. (Psalm 88:9)

Whenever we keep ourselves back from doing the work that we should, our hands may be affected.

Putting forth our hands for harm

One of the ways in which we keep ourselves from doing good is by doing things we shouldn't. A notable character who put out his hand for evil in the Old Testament is Jeroboam.

> And it came to pass, when king Jeroboam heard the saying of the man of God, which had cried against the altar in Bethel, that he put forth his hand from the altar, saying, Lay hold on him. And his hand, which he put forth against him, dried up, so that he could not pull it in again to him. (1 Kings 13:4)

Because he used his hand for an evil purpose, God caused it to dry up.

When we start to spend our time in inappropriate activities, rather than in the Lord's work, we may suffer problems with our hands. We may have a particular interest that takes up our time and stops us being fully involved in the Lord's work *(see also bottom of page 48,* What about injury?). Paul says,

> I beseech you therefore, brethren, by the mercies of God, that ye present your bodies a living sacrifice, holy, acceptable unto God, which is your reasonable service. (Romans 12:1)

Wrong attitudes towards fellow-workers

In biblical times, as today, to shake hands (or *strike* hands), was a sign of friendship and good will. We see this in operation in Galatians:

> And when James, Cephas, and John, who seemed to be pillars, perceived the grace that was given unto me, they gave to me and Barnabas the right hands of fellowship; that we should go unto the heathen, and they unto the circumcision. (Galatians 2:9)

Inasmuch as different parts of the physical body represent different parts of the body of Christ, (the church), a wrong attitude towards certain parts of the church can bring illness to our bodies (I Corinthians 12). The hands represent the workers in the church, so when we have a pain in our hands it can be because we have unloving attitudes towards our fellow-workers. In normal circumstances, most people in the local assembly will count as fellow-workers.

Arm

Since the arm provides the power behind the hand, it symbolises the strength of a person to act, to accomplish something. When Mary magnifies the Lord in song, she speaks of His power:

> He hath shewed strength with his arm. (Luke 1:51)

She then recites a list of great things that the Lord has done in demonstration of His might. It is the arm that is said to be the strength behind the actions.

An injured or diseased arm indicates something is causing us to lose our strength to act.

Thumb

Inasmuch as the thumb leads the rest of the hand, it speaks especially of our leadership and direction in the realm of our work.

Nails

Nails protect our fingers, and speak of the way in which we protect our fellow-workers. A damaged nail indicates we are failing to protect our co-workers. An in-growing nail indicates that rather than protecting them we are actually harming them.

Way of healing

We may find that we are very inefficient when it comes to spiritual work. We may prefer to do things other than the work of God, particularly in our spare time. We may prefer to please ourselves rather than to please God. We may be slow to get on with the work God has given us, perhaps through laziness.

Our inefficiency may be increased by our poor attitude towards our fellow workers. For a workforce to work well together, its members must be in agreement and work together.

Confess that you have allowed things to become obstacles to the work you should be doing for God. See the importance of being utterly committed to serving Christ.

Helpful scriptures

I Corinthians 7:29-31; Philippians 3:7-17; Romans 13:11-14; Romans 12:1-2

Head (*see also* <u>Neurological</u>)

Spiritual meaning: relationship to authority

Scriptures
- I would have you know, that the head of every man is Christ; and the head of the woman is the man; and the head of Christ is God. (I Corinthians 11:3)
- The centurion answered and said, Lord, I am not worthy that thou shouldest come under my roof: but speak the word only, and my servant shall be healed. For I am a man under authority, having soldiers under me: and I say to this man, Go, and he goeth; and to another, Come, and he cometh; and to my servant, Do this, and he doeth it. (Matthew 8:8-9)

Explanation of connection
The head speaks to us of authority. The authority that a person has comes not from himself but from the one that is over him, that is, his 'head'. Christ is the 'head' of the church, meaning He is in authority over it (Ephesians 5:23). The Bible says that Christ is under the authority of God the Father, that the man is under the authority of Christ, and the woman is under the authority of the man. Therefore, when we act on our own authority or fail to respect and submit to authority, we are damaging our head. For a woman to usurp authority over her husband is to damage her head. For a man to act on his own authority rather than under the authority of Christ is to damage his head.

The one who, in the Bible, most obviously tried to usurp the place of God was Satan. For this reason, the Bible says, his head would be crushed. In the garden of Eden, God says to the serpent,

And I will put enmity between thee and the woman, and between thy seed and her seed; it shall bruise thy head, and thou shalt bruise his heel. (Genesis 3:15)

Therefore when our physical head is affected by illness or pain, such as a headache, it is an indication that we are failing to submit to authority. That authority may be a human, or it may be God himself.

The Bible tells us that all authority is from God.

Let every soul be subject unto the higher powers. For there is no power but of God: the powers that be are ordained of God. Whosoever therefore resisteth the power, resisteth the ordinance of God: and they that resist shall receive to themselves damnation. (Romans 13:1-2)

Therefore we should be always in subjection to those over us, whether it be the government of the country, our parents, those over us at work, our teachers, our church leadership, or the police.

For rulers are not a terror to good works, but to the evil. Wilt thou then not be afraid of the power? do that which is good, and thou shalt have praise of the same: for he is the minister of God to thee for good. But if thou do that which is evil, be afraid; for he beareth not the sword in vain: for he is the minister of God, a revenger to execute wrath upon him that doeth evil. Wherefore ye must needs be subject, not only for wrath, but also for conscience sake. For for this cause pay ye tribute also: for they are God's ministers, attending continually upon this very thing. Render therefore to all their dues: tribute to whom tribute is due; custom to whom custom; fear to whom fear; honour to whom honour. (Romans 13:3-7)

The only time when one can go against authority is when a higher authority orders you to do so. Therefore, if an authority orders you to disobey God, you must submit to God rather than man.

Then Peter and the other apostles answered and said, We ought to obey God rather than men. (Acts 5:29)

Thinking in our own strength

One of the ways in which we cease to submit to authority is by trying to work things out for ourselves, by thinking in our own strength, rather than allowing Christ to be in control and to reveal things to us. This too can cause pains to the head.

Way of healing
Admit that you have been acting on your own authority. You have taken it upon yourself to be the final authority rather than being in subjection to God and those above you. Confess this and ask for your healing.

Helpful scriptures
Philippians 2:5-11; I Peter 2:11-25; I Timothy 2:12; Hebrews 7:7, 17

Heart

Spiritual meaning: relates to how one's life is driven

Scriptures
- Whither shall we go up? our brethren have discouraged [or *wasted with illness*] our heart, saying, The people is greater and taller than we. (Deuteronomy 1:28)
- Give therefore thy servant an understanding heart to judge thy people, that I may discern between good and bad: for who is able to judge this thy so great a people? (I Kings 3:9)
- He that is slow to wrath is of great understanding: but he that is hasty of spirit exalteth folly. A sound heart is the life of the flesh: but envy the rottenness of the bones. (Proverbs 14:29, 30)
- The heart is deceitful above all things, and desperately wicked: who can know it? (Jeremiah 17:9)
- Every man according as he purposeth in his heart, so let him give; not grudgingly, or of necessity: for God loveth a cheerful giver. (II Corinthians 9:7)

Explanation of connection
In the physical body, the heart is the organ that pumps blood around the body; it is the organ that drives our bodies. Since

blood represents a person's *life* (Leviticus 17:11), the spiritual heart is that part of us which drives us, which drives our lives. It may loosely be described as our will.

It can be affected by many different things but ultimately makes up its own mind. It may be informed by the brain but may choose not to listen. It may choose to be guided by God. It may respond to other people.

When something happens to us, the heart responds. If it is a bad thing that has happened, the heart, our driving force, may be troubled and discouraged. We may in such circumstances lose the will to live or to keep going in something. Because our will is the part of us that is affected by circumstances and events, the heart is also the seat of the emotions.

Since it is the part of us that drives us and responds to things, it is the place where ultimate decisions and judgements are made. If the heart is not in something, the rest of the person has to bow to it.

When we have a good heart, it responds to things in the right way. A bad heart will respond corruptly, a hard heart will be unresponsive and stubborn, a discouraged heart will be weak or faint, and a strong heart will be bold and courageous.

Arrhythmias

Problems with the heart rate or rhythm may be caused by driving your life to the wrong rhythm. A fast heart beat indicates that you are moving too fast, perhaps getting over-excited, het up, or stressed. An excessively slow rate will indicate being too laid back and relaxed. An irregular pattern may indicate changeability in the spiritual heart, perhaps between the two extremes.

Angina and Coronary Thrombosis

As an organ, the physical heart, as well as pumping the blood, needs its own supply of blood. When an artery carrying blood to the heart becomes narrow or blocked, the heart does not get sufficient oxygen and nutrients. Angina is the pain caused by the restricted flow of blood. A thrombosis is a blockage to the supply.

In our spiritual lives, we sometimes get very concerned about trivial things. This is like not giving our heart its proper supply of blood, the life that it needs in order to be effective. We get interested in and spend time on things that are of no real value and consequence. We may get very bothered about small amounts of money. We get het up and angry over small things. We may be mean-spirited, not wanting others to have things, such as success. All these are different examples of what is known as being 'small-minded' but might better be described as 'narrow-hearted'.

If we spend much time worrying about trivia rather than the big things of life we may get angina, a narrowing of the flow of life. If we suddenly get extremely worked up and dominated by trivial things, perhaps one thing in particular, it may cause a thrombosis. Our hearts and wills should be fed by the life of Christ to remain effective and healthy.

Hypertrophic cardiomyopathy, Hardened arteries (relates to angina above)

Pharaoh is possibly the best example of someone with a hard heart in the Bible. When God told him repeatedly to release the children of Israel from Egypt, he refused. Even when he was seeing the most remarkable miracles and when he and his country were being plagued, he would not obey God. His will was unbending, his heart was hard:

> And when Pharaoh saw that the rain and the hail and the thunders were ceased, he sinned yet more, and hardened his heart, he and his servants. And the heart of Pharaoh was hardened, neither would he let the children of Israel go; as the LORD had spoken by Moses. (Exodus 9:34, 35)

The Lord Jesus in contrast is described as 'meek and lowly in heart' (Matthew 11:29), with the word for meek meaning *soft* and *gentle,* and therefore responsive.

A healthy physical heart should be both strong to pump the blood, yet supple so that it allows a free flow of blood. In the physical, a thickened heart and hardened coronary arteries limit the flow of blood through the heart and to the heart, causing a heart attack, angina and other symptoms. In the spiritual, if we are hard hearted and stubborn, we are limiting the flow of life to and through our lives. It will be noted that Pharaoh was not only stubborn, but his stubbornness also showed itself in meanness – he would not let the Hebrews have what was due to them.

Heart Attack

A restriction of the coronary arteries may cause a heart attack, in which part of the heart dies. This obviously represents the fact that the spiritual heart has been so deprived of life, through mean-spiritedness etc., that it has partially ceased to function altogether.

Heart failure

In various places in scripture it speaks of people's hearts failing them. An example of this is found in Genesis when Joseph's brothers have been to visit him as Prime Minister of Egypt to buy corn. When they discover that they still have the money that they thought they had handed over, they are left lifeless.

> And he said unto his brethren, My money is restored; and, lo, it is even in my sack: and their heart failed them, and they were afraid, saying one to another, What is this that God hath done unto us? (Genesis 42:28)

When things in life become too much for us, when we are put under excessive pressure, we can become so afraid that our hearts fail us. We simply do not have the strength or courage to keep going and we lose our will to continue. The physical heart follows the will in becoming weak or giving up altogether.

Dilated cardiomyopathy

If the heart grows too large, it becomes weak. This indicates being too broad-minded. Spiritually, if we are too big-hearted, accepting everything and judging nothing, too indulgent and generous, our drive in life may become weak.

Endocarditis

A bacterial or fungal infection of the heart, which comes through the blood from another source, may indicate that the spiritual heart has been affected from sin in another area of a person's life. For example, a bitter attitude might so affect a person that his drive in life is affected.

Hole in the heart

A *hole in the heart* is a hole between the right and left atria of the heart. De-oxygenated blood enters the heart into the right atrium. It then moves into the right ventricle which pumps it to the lungs. Oxygenated blood returns into the left atrium before going into the left ventricle which pumps it round the whole body.

A. Right to left shunt

When someone has a hole in the heart, de-oxygenated blood can move directly from the right atrium to the left without going via the lungs and getting oxygen. This indicates someone is trying to drive their lives on without going to God for the empowering and energising of the Holy Spirit.

B. Left to right shunt

Alternatively, oxygenated blood can move back from the left to right atrium, where it is pumped to the lungs a second time. This means that a person continually seeks to improve their spiritual life, to receive the infilling of the Holy Spirit, without then driving their life on to act in His power.

For information on the implications of a hole in the heart's being a congenital condition, please see congenital disorders, *page 141.*

General principles of blood-flow related diseases

When the blood flows back, it indicates a lack of drive. When the blood does not reach the lungs, it indicates that that person is not allowing their life to be oxygenated by the Holy Spirit. Oxygenated blood which is prevented from leaving the heart indicates a life that is oxygenated by the Holy Spirit but not released in action, service etc; it is not outworked.

Way of healing

The Bible says that 'The heart is deceitful above all things, and desperately wicked: who can know it?' (Jeremiah 17:9). The word translated 'desperately wicked' literally means 'incurable'. It is naturally corrupt because of sin. It will naturally always make the wrong choice, it will choose to rebel against God, whilst at the same time fooling itself that it is doing right (hence *deceitful*). For this reason, it is no good repairing the spiritual heart: it has to be replaced.

> A new heart also will I give you, and a new spirit will I put within you: and I will take away the stony heart out of your flesh, and I will give you an heart of flesh. And I will put my spirit within you, and cause you to walk in my statutes, and ye shall keep my judgments, and do them. (Ezekiel 36:26, 27)

We need, therefore, to come to God and ask Him to give us a new heart. When we were saved we were given a new heart, but as we go on in our spiritual lives, we often start to take back the old stony heart of the old nature. Confess that your heart is corrupt and asking the Lord to give you His heart. Confess the areas particularly where your heart is wrong as outlined above.

Helpful scriptures
Arrhythmias
John 15:1-11
Faint heart
Psalm 27; John 14:1-3; Joshua 1:7; Psalm 31
Angina, Coronary Thrombosis, Heart Attack
Philippians 2:5-11; Deuteronomy 30:19

Hernia

Spiritual cause: moving out of your sphere of service

Scriptures
- Jesus Christ himself being the chief corner stone; in whom all the building fitly framed together groweth unto an holy temple in the Lord. (Ephesians 20-21)
- For the body is not one member, but many. If the foot shall

say, Because I am not the hand, I am not of the body; is it
therefore not of the body? And if the ear shall say, Because
I am not the eye, I am not of the body; is it therefore not
of the body? If the whole body were an eye, where were
the hearing? If the whole were hearing, where were the
smelling? But now hath God set the members every one
of them in the body, as it hath pleased him. (I Corinthians
12:14-18)

Explanation of connection

In physical terms a hernia is when an internal organ protrudes
out of the area enclosing it. In spiritual terms, it speaks of when
we have moved outside the area of service that God has allotted
to us.

The Bible says that the church is like a body: it is made up of
many different parts, each with its own particular role to play. In
order for the church to be effective, each member has to do the
work that God has given to him.

Christ: From whom the whole body fitly joined together and
compacted by that which every joint supplieth, according to
the effectual working in the measure of every part, maketh
increase of the body unto the edifying of itself in love.
(Ephesians 4:16)

If each member plays its allotted role, the whole body is healthy
and effective, everyone's needs are met, and the body is able to
grow.

Sometimes, however, we feel that we want to do something
else. We grow tired of our work and want to take over someone
else's work. We may, for example, be called to run the recording
system in the local assembly. However, we may begin to think
we should have a more prominent role, that our real calling is as
a Bible teacher. We try, therefore to jettison our work and seize
every opportunity to preach.

This causes a series of problems. It prevents us from doing our
own work properly. It means we start to encroach on someone
else's area of service. We may get in their way, and make their

work more difficult. We may find ourselves criticising the way they are doing their work, because we feel we would do it better.

We may also decide to leave our church, and seek another church where we think we will be more 'used' – where we can do the job we are coveting. Again, that is moving out of the place God has called us to.

However, we need to see that Christ is the head of the church. It is His church and He must decide the role that each part of the body must play.

Way of healing

Admit that you have not been content to play the part God has given to you, that you have moved or tried to move out of the place in which God has put you, perhaps that you have encroached into someone else's sphere of service. Seek from the Lord exactly where He wants you and what He wants you to do. Then ask for your healing.

Helpful scriptures

Philippians 2:3; 4:11-12; Jeremiah 45:5; Ecclesiastes 9:10

Hip

Spiritual meaning: submission to God

Scriptures

- And when he saw that he prevailed not against him, he touched the hollow of his thigh; and the hollow of Jacob's thigh was out of joint, as he wrestled with him. (Genesis 32:25)

Explanation of connection

The hip joint is the strongest joint in the human body. It is also the central pivot of the whole body. Traditionally it was the place where the sword was worn (Psalm 45:3). In spiritual terms, our hip joint speaks of the issue in our lives on which we are most unwilling to submit, and which God wants to deal with the most. It is the central factor in our spiritual lives.

We see this in the case of Jacob. God was wanting to deal with the major problem in his life, his propensity to try to get everything in life by his own cunning rather than trusting God for them. For a long time he will not submit to God, he will not respond. Finally God decides that the issue cannot go on any longer, and must be dealt with. God wrestles with Jacob, and when Jacob will not give in God strikes his thigh, the strongest part of him, so that he has to submit to God. *(For more on this passage, see* Chapter 10: The day of Jacob's Trouble, *page 74).*

When we are suffering with hip problems, it means that God is trying to deal with a defining issue in our lives and we are not responding and submitting. It will very often coincide with another illness which speaks of the specific issue on which we won't submit. God is saying, I don't want you to go any further until this issue is dealt with.

Explanation of cause/way of healing
Realize that God is seeking to deal with the central problem in your spiritual life. Confess to Him your unwillingness to submit, and seek Him to know what He wants to deal with.

Helpful scriptures
Matthew 5:25; James 4:6-10; Psalm 100:3

Homosexuality

Spiritual cause: **Vanity/self love**

Scriptures
- Professing themselves to be wise, they became fools, And changed the glory of the uncorruptible God into an image made like to corruptible man, and to birds, and fourfooted beasts, and creeping things. Wherefore God also gave them up to uncleanness through the lusts of

their own hearts, to dishonour their own bodies between themselves: who changed the truth of God into a lie, and worshipped and served the creature more than the Creator, who is blessed for ever. Amen. For this cause God gave them up unto vile affections: for even their women did change the natural use into that which is against nature: and likewise also the men, leaving the natural use of the woman, burned in their lust one toward another; men with men working that which is unseemly, and receiving in themselves that recompence of their error which was meet. (Romans 1:26, 27).

Explanation of connection

If a person has a high opinion of himself, he will become vain. He has turned himself into his own idol, has fallen in love with himself and has started worshipping himself. When this reaches an extreme, he becomes attracted to people exactly like himself: to carry this through to its final conclusion, that means people of the same gender.

The truth of this is seen in the link between homosexuality and vanity regarding personal appearance. Viewing oneself more than necessary in the mirror is a typical symptom of this and will exacerbate it.

The biblical example of this is clear in Romans 1. A people who have rejected God begin to worship the creature rather than the creator. They have replaced God with a human image and started to worship that. In response God says that He gave such people up to the extreme sin of homosexuality.

Way of healing

Confess that you have made an idol of yourself and failed to see God as He really is – the glorious resplendent eternal God who has created the world for His glory. Confess that you haven't worshipped God as the only true God. Make Him your all in all and He will heal you of your vanity.

Helpful scriptures

Leviticus 18:22; I Timothy 2:5; Exodus 20:3-6

Immune system

Spiritual meaning: conscience

Scriptures
- Submit yourselves therefore to God. Resist the devil, and he will flee from you. (James 4:7)
- Ye have not yet resisted unto blood, striving against sin. (Hebrews 12:4)
- Put on the whole armour of God, that ye may be able to stand against the wiles of the devil. For we wrestle not against flesh and blood, but against principalities, against powers, against the rulers of the darkness of this world, against spiritual wickedness in high places. Wherefore take unto you the whole armour of God, that ye may be able to withstand in the evil day, and having done all, to stand. (Ephesians 6:11-13)
- Be sober, be vigilant; because your adversary the devil, as a roaring lion, walketh about, seeking whom he may devour: Whom resist stedfast in the faith, knowing that the same afflictions are accomplished in your brethren that are in the world. (I Peter 5:8-9)

Explanation
In the physical, our immune system recognizes, resists and deals with *pathogens* – those bacteria and viruses that enter our bodies and cause disease.

The spiritual parallel to the immune system is our ability to recognize resist and deal with evil. The heart of our spiritual immune system depends on our conscience and our knowledge of God.

In Romans 1 it talks about a people who have dismissed God from their consciousness.

That which may be known of God is manifest in them; for God hath shewed it unto them. For the invisible things of him from the creation of the world are clearly seen, being understood by the things that are made, even his eternal power and Godhead; so that they are without excuse: because that, when they knew God, they glorified him not as God, neither were thankful; but became vain in their imaginations, and their foolish heart was darkened. Professing themselves to be wise, they became fools, and changed the glory of the uncorruptible God into an image made like to corruptible man, and to birds, and fourfooted beasts, and creeping things. (Romans 1:19-23)

Because they have removed all thoughts of God from their minds and let their conscience die, they have lost their ability to resist evil. Consequently, they fall into sin.

And even as they did not like to retain God in their knowledge, God gave them over to a reprobate mind, to do those things which are not convenient; being filled with all unrighteousness, fornication, wickedness, covetousness, maliciousness; full of envy, murder, debate, deceit, malignity; whisperers, backbiters, haters of God, despiteful, proud, boasters, inventors of evil things, disobedient to parents, without understanding, covenantbreakers, without natural affection, implacable, unmerciful: who knowing the judgment of God, that they which commit such things are worthy of death, not only do the same, but have pleasure in them that do them. (Romans I:28-32)

Someone whose immune system is not working has so neglected God and let their conscience die that they can no longer tell when something is wrong and resist evil. Consequently, they commit sins which in turn bring disease upon the body. That's what the passage means by 'receiving in themselves that recompence of their error which was meet.'

HIV/AIDS

HIV is a disease that destroys the immune system. Thus, when an HIV positive person is invaded by a pathogen (such as a virus), they are unable to deal with it. This demonstrates that, in spiritual terms, through removing God from their consciousness, their conscience has been destroyed. Thus, when sin and temptation come along, they are unable to deal with them.

The fact that HIV is especially spread amongst people who commit the sins highlighted in Romans 1, particularly fornication and homosexuality, emphasises the connection. A person may contract HIV through other means, such as receiving contaminated blood. Yet, in such cases, their illness will still indicate a lack of conscience in the person, even if they didn't contract HIV from sinful activity.

When a child inherits HIV from its mother, it is God saying that, unless the next generation turns to God, it will follow in the sins of the parents (*see also* What about children, *page 53*).

For this reason, when HIV/AIDS is rife in a country, what the people need above all things is the gospel and the truth of God.

Spleen

The spleen's function is to filter the blood and remove bacteria and viruses, and to remove old red blood cells. The spleen therefore speaks of a person's discernment, their ability to detect and remove harmful things from their lives. Discernment also enables a person to lay aside old spiritual experiences so that a new experience and revelation can be enjoyed.

Tonsils

The tonsils are part of the immune system and operate in the throat. Being situated behind the mouth and along the respiratory tract, the tonsils speak of our conscience with regard to our thoughts and words. If our tonsils have become infected, it means we are not careful about what we think and say.

How healing comes

Confess to God that you have dismissed Him from your thoughts and allowed your conscience to become weak. You can then ask for your healing.

Obviously, there may be other sins that have been committed because of your weak conscience which have brought other diseases. Confess these and receive your healing for each disease.

Infectious diseases

Spiritual meaning: sin caused by our response to the sins of other people

Scriptures
- Be not deceived: evil communications corrupt good manners. (I Corinthians 15:33)
- Lay hands suddenly on no man, neither be partaker of other men's sins: keep thyself pure. (I Timothy 5:22)

Explanation of connection
An infectious disease is caused by a *pathogen* (virus, bacteria etc.) entering a person's body. Infectious diseases can be transmitted from person to person in different ways: by inhaling droplets of saliva, through food and water, and through other agents such as mosquitoes.

Infectious diseases speak of our response to the sins of other people. For example, when a person is rude, we may respond to them either by loving them or hating them. If we respond to their sin by sinning ourselves, we have been infected by it. Equally, if we are influenced by other people and start committing the sins they commit, we have been infected by their sins.

Influenza, common cold, Mumps, Rubella, Measles (*see also* <u>Colds and Fevers,</u> <u>Rash</u> as appropriate)
These diseases are all transmitted by droplets of fluid from an infected person's nose and mouth being inhaled by another person. Since *water* symbolises *words,* it indicates that a person is sinning as a result of their response to the words of another person.

Smallpox, Chicken pox, shingles
Inasmuch as these diseases affect the <u>skin,</u> they indicate pride coming as a response to the sins of others.

Way of healing

Confess that you have sinned in response to the sins of other people. Identify the specific sins, confess them to the Lord, and ask for your healing.

Helpful scriptures

Matthew 7:1; Romans 2:1-4

Itching (pruritus)

Spiritual cause: discontent

Scriptures

- For the time will come when they will not listen to the sound doctrine, but, having itching ears, will heap up for themselves teachers after their own lusts; and will turn away their ears from the truth, and turn aside to fables. (II Timothy 4:3-4)

Explanation of connection

When we have an itch, an area of our body feels uncomfortable and discontent: it wants to be scratched. This speaks in the spiritual of discontent in an aspect of our lives. For example, when we feel discontent and want to go somewhere else, we may have itchy feet. If we wish we were doing a different job, we may get itchy hands. *(Please see the part of the body affected under its own heading, or consult* Quick Reference, *page 114)*.

In the passage quoted above, the people in question are discontent with the sound teaching that they are getting, and require something more satisfying to the flesh.

Way of healing

Confess that you have been discontent in an area of your life, and ask for your healing.

Helpful scriptures

Philippians 4:10-12; I Timothy 6; Matthew 6:19-34

Kidneys

Spiritual meaning: relates to the things that guide you

Scriptures

- I will bless the LORD, who hath given me counsel: my **reins** also instruct me in the night seasons. (Psalm 16:7)
- Judge me, O LORD; for I have walked in mine integrity: I have trusted also in the LORD; therefore I shall not slide. Examine me, O LORD, and prove me; try my **reins** and my heart. (Psalm 26:1, 2)
- Thus my heart was grieved, and I was pricked in my **reins**. So foolish was I, and ignorant: I was as a beast before thee. Nevertheless I am continually with thee: thou hast holden me by my right hand. Thou shalt guide me with thy counsel, and afterward receive me to glory. (Psalm 73:21-24)

Explanation of connection

Throughout the Bible, in both the Old Testament and the New, the word translated as *reins* is the word *kidneys* (indeed in old-fashioned English *reins* is another word for kidneys). Reins are what we use to steer a horse. Therefore our kidneys symbolise our spiritual reins, the way in which our lives are guided and controlled. In order for our lives to be controlled properly, our reins need to be wholly put into God's hands. We need to be directed by Him.

In physical terms, the kidneys are the part of the body that filters waste from our blood: they choose what stays and what is removed from the blood. Since *blood* represents *life* (*see* <u>Blood</u>) this speaks of our faculty of choosing what is good and should remain in our lives, and what is bad and should be removed. Again, it is a kind of guide and control.

Sometimes, however, this faculty becomes corrupted and we guide our lives in the flesh: since we are not letting God hold our reins we let the wrong things remain in our lives. We may use our own intellect and ideas to guide us. We may be influenced by our own fleshly desires. We may be led by the popular ideas of the day. We may follow the ways of the world, listening to philosophers, psychologists and other secular theorists. We may get our guidance from newspapers, magazines, the television and radio.

Kidneys that are diseased indicate that our spiritual reins have become impaired and corrupted: our lives are not being filtered to remove what is bad. God calls us to be guided entirely by Him, to have the mind of Christ. This is only possible if we cease to listen to all these other voices and commit ourselves to seeking His face through prayer and reading His written word, the Bible.

Way of healing
Confess that you have not been allowing God to guide your life. You have been controlling your life in the flesh. Be willing to be guided and influenced entirely by the Lord. Then ask for your healing.

Helpful scriptures
Proverbs 3:1-12; Romans 12:2

Knee

Spiritual meaning: relates to strength and prayer

Scriptures
- All hands shall be feeble, and all knees shall be weak as water. (Ezekiel 7:17)
- So he brought down the people unto the water: and the LORD said unto Gideon, Every one that lappeth of the water with his tongue, as a dog lappeth, him shalt thou set by himself; likewise every one that boweth down upon his knees to drink. And the number of them that lapped, putting their hand to their mouth, were three hundred men: but all the rest of the people bowed down upon their knees to drink water. (Judges 7:5, 6)
- And she made him sleep upon her knees; and she called for a man, and she caused him to shave off the seven locks of his head; and she began to afflict him, and his strength went from him. (Judges 16:19)

- Strengthen ye the weak hands, and confirm the feeble knees. Say to them that are of a fearful heart, Be strong, fear not: behold, your God will come with vengeance, even God with a recompence; he will come and save you. (Isaiah 35:3, 4)

Explanation of connection

In different ways throughout the Bible, the knees are used to speak of weakness. When we are feeble or weak, it is said to be the knees that go weak.

And it shall be, when they say unto thee, Wherefore sighest thou? that thou shalt answer, For the tidings; because it cometh: and every heart shall melt, and all hands shall be feeble, and every spirit shall faint, and all knees shall be weak as water: behold, it cometh, and shall be brought to pass, saith the Lord GOD. (Ezekiel 21:7)

Equally, when we fall on our knees before someone, it shows our weakness before them and therefore our humility and submission. When a man came to Jesus whose sick son even the disciples could not heal, he is in a state of utter dependency and weakness: he can do absolutely nothing about the situation himself and he shows it by kneeling before Jesus.

And when they were come to the multitude, there came to him a certain man, kneeling down to him, and saying, Lord, have mercy on my son: for he is lunatick, and sore vexed: for ofttimes he falleth into the fire, and oft into the water. (Matthew 17:14-15)

Therefore, if we are suffering with weak or problematic physical knees, it means we are being weak in the spiritual realm

What is interesting, however, is the way in which we deal with our weakness. The Bible makes it clear that our strength comes from God, and that we receive His strength by acknowledging our weakness before Him. The Apostle Paul says of the Lord,

And he said unto me, My grace is sufficient for thee: for my strength is made perfect in weakness. Most gladly therefore will I rather glory in my infirmities, that the power of Christ may rest upon me. Therefore I take pleasure in infirmities, in reproaches, in necessities, in persecutions, in distresses for Christ's sake: for when I am weak, then am I strong. (II Corinthians 12:9-10)

It is therefore by kneeling before God that we receive our strength. For this reason, prayer lies at the heart of spiritual strength. It says in Isaiah 'they that wait upon the LORD shall renew their strength' (Isaiah 40:31).

Kneeling is biblically very much a part of submissive prayer, together with lifting up of hands before God:

And at the evening sacrifice I arose up from my heaviness; and having rent my garment and my mantle, I fell upon my knees, and spread out my hands unto the LORD my God. (Ezra 9:5 – see also I Kings 8:54)

Therefore, when it says 'lift up the hands which hang down, and the feeble knees' (Hebrews 12:12), it really means, strengthen your spiritual attitude, and do so by humble fervent prayer before God.

Way of healing
See that you have become spiritually weak, and that this is because your prayer life has been lacking. Confess it before God. Strengthen yourself in prayer, and ask for your physical healing.

Labour pains (childbirth)

Spiritual cause: relates to holiness

Scriptures
- Unto the woman he said, I will greatly multiply thy sorrow and thy conception; in sorrow thou shalt bring forth children; and thy desire shall be to thy husband, and he shall rule over thee. (Genesis 3:16)

- Let the woman learn in silence with all subjection. But I suffer not a woman to teach, nor to usurp authority over the man, but to be in silence. For Adam was first formed, then Eve. And Adam was not deceived, but the woman being deceived was in the transgression. Notwithstanding she shall be saved [*preserved*] in childbearing, if they continue in faith and charity and holiness with sobriety. (I Timothy 2:11-15)

Explanation of connection

In scripture, the concept of labour (travail) in giving birth is closely associated with fear. In Jeremiah 30, when Judah was about to go into captivity, the prophet speaks of the fear that will come upon the men when they are faced with a conquering enemy which they can do nothing about. This fear is described as that of a woman in labour.

> For thus saith the LORD; We have heard a voice of trembling, of fear, and not of peace. Ask ye now, and see whether a man doth travail with child? wherefore do I see every man with his hands on his loins, as a woman in travail, and all faces are turned into paleness? Alas! for that day is great, so that none is like it: it is even the time of Jacob's trouble, but he shall be saved out of it. (Jeremiah 30:5-7)

The reason is this: because the people were not right with God, when the enemy attacked, they knew they could not expect God to do anything about it; he was no longer their defence.

We see the same thing in the garden of Eden. Adam and Eve had always had a relationship of trust and friendship with God. However, when they eat of the forbidden fruit, for the first time they are afraid of God.

> And he [Adam] said, I heard thy voice in the garden, and I was afraid, because I was naked; and I hid myself. (Genesis 3:10)

It is soon after this that God says in response to the woman's disobedience:

> I will greatly multiply thy sorrow and thy conception; in sorrow thou shalt bring forth children; and thy desire shall be to thy husband, and he shall rule over thee. (Genesis 3:16)

The reason that the woman took and ate the fruit in the first place was because she had no reverential fear for God. When she has to face God having sinned, she feels fear, but it is the fear that comes from shame. In consequence she is told that she will suffer pain in childbirth.

When a woman is giving birth, she is naked before God. It is perhaps the most important thing that she will have to do in life, and the most difficult. For this reason, she is utterly at the mercy of God and needs to be able utterly to depend upon Him. If she has a good conscience, if she is walking in godliness before God, she will not be afraid in the time of her trouble. She will be like Adam and Eve before they sinned, who were 'both naked, the man and his wife, and were not ashamed.' She knows that God will be there to help her and will give an easy delivery. If she is not right with God, in the day of her trouble she will know that she cannot expect God to come to her aid.

> For Adam was first formed, then Eve. And Adam was not deceived, but the woman being deceived was in the transgression. Notwithstanding she shall be saved [preserved] in childbearing, if they continue in faith and charity and holiness with sobriety. (I Timothy 2:14-15)

A major issue in a woman living a godly life is to be in right relationship to her husband. Throughout scripture women are told to be in submission to their husbands.

> Likewise, ye wives, be in subjection to your own husbands; that, if any obey not the word, they also may without the word be won by the conversation [lifestyle] of the wives. (I Peter 3:1)

This will be an important part of 'holiness with sobriety'.

In referring to the re-establishing of the state of Israel, God describes it as giving birth. It is interesting to note, however, that the message is addressed to those that have godly fear:

Hear the word of the LORD, ye that tremble at his word; your brethren that hated you, that cast you out for my name's sake, said, Let the LORD be glorified: but he shall appear to your joy, and they shall be ashamed. Before she travailed, she brought forth; before her pain came, she was delivered of a man child. Who hath heard such a thing? who hath seen such things? Shall the earth be made to bring forth in one day? or shall a nation be born at once? for as soon as Zion travailed, she brought forth her children. Shall I bring to the birth, and not cause to bring forth? saith the LORD: shall I cause to bring forth, and shut the womb? saith thy God. (Isaiah 66:5, 7-9)

Menstrual pains *(see also* Reproductive System, Female*)*

Menstrual pains indicate the woman is living in a way that is harmful to her (future) role of childbearing. This may include a bad attitude to childbearing or an aspect of it. *See also* Menorrhoea.

Way of healing

In order to give birth without fear of pain, it is necessary to be utterly right with God. Spend time seeking His face to know if there is anything in your life that is displeasing to Him. Make use of Finney on *Breaking up the Fallow Ground,* page 92. Be ready for labour with a completely clear conscience and there will be nothing to fear.

Helpful scriptures

II Chronicles 20:1-28

Liver

Spiritual meaning: **honour**

Scriptures

- Dead flies cause the ointment of the apothecary to send forth a stinking savour: so doth a little folly him that is in reputation for wisdom and **honour**. Ecclesiastes 10:1
- And I will yet be more vile than thus, and will be base in mine own sight: and of the maidservants which thou hast

spoken of, of them shall I be had in **honour**. (II Samuel 6:22)

- Both riches and **honour** come of thee, and thou reignest over all; and in thine hand is power and might; and in thine hand it is to make great, and to give strength unto all. (I Chronicles 29:12)
- *See also* Psalm 7:4-5; Proverbs 26:1, 8

Explanation of connection

The word for *liver* in Hebrew comes from the word with the basic meaning *to be heavy* (the liver is the heaviest organ). The root of the word for *liver* is widely translated *to be honourable* – that is, to be a person of weight, a person of substance. When we devote our lives to things that are weighty and serious, and we take God seriously, we become people of honour. When we fail to take God seriously and live foolishly, we become dishonourable. **A diseased liver indicates a lack of honour in a person's life.**

God says that the way in which we become honourable is by showing honour to Him. This is made clear in His dealings with Eli the priest. God reproaches Eli for the way in which he has dealt with his sons, taking no trouble to correct them when they are behaving wickedly. He particularly rebukes him for honouring his sons more than God.

> Wherefore kick ye at my sacrifice and at mine offering, which I have commanded in my habitation; and honourest thy sons above me, to make yourselves fat with the chiefest of all the offerings of Israel my people? (I Samuel 2:29)

God says that the consequence of Eli's not honouring Him is that Eli himself will lose his honour.

> Wherefore the LORD God of Israel saith, I said indeed that thy house, and the house of thy father, should walk before me for ever: but now the LORD saith, Be it far from me; for them that honour me I will honour, and they that despise me shall be lightly esteemed. (I Samuel 2:30)

It is not surprising, therefore, that a person who drinks heavily will become dishonourable – they have not been honouring God. Their lives will fall apart, they will behave dishonourably, and ultimately this will be manifest in a damaged liver.

> Thou art filled with shame for glory: drink thou also, and let thy foreskin be uncovered: the cup of the LORD's right hand shall be turned unto thee, and shameful spewing shall be on thy glory [or *honour*]. (Habakkuk 2:16)

A person's honour or dishonour depends on whether they live wisely or foolishly, and the Bible many times connects honour with wisdom. When Solomon asked not for honour, but for wisdom from God, God in return gives him riches and honour as well as wisdom.

> Behold, I have done according to thy words: lo, I have given thee a wise and an understanding heart; so that there was none like thee before thee, neither after thee shall any arise like unto thee. And I have also given thee that which thou hast not asked, both riches, and honour: so that there shall not be any among the kings like unto thee all thy days. (I Kings 3:12-13)

The Psalmist says,

> The fear of the LORD is the beginning of wisdom: a good understanding have all they that do his commandments: his praise endureth for ever. (Psalm 111:10)

Therefore, if we honour God in our lives and obey Him, we will have wisdom and be able to live honourably. Different people whose good actions indicate that they honour God in scripture are described as honourable:

- A gracious woman retaineth honour. (Proverbs 11:16)
- It is an honour for a man to cease from strife: but every fool will be meddling. (Proverbs 20:3)
- Poverty and shame shall be to him that refuseth instruction:

but he that regardeth reproof shall be honoured. (Proverbs 13:18)
- The fear of the LORD is the instruction of wisdom; and before honour is humility. (Proverbs 15:33)
- A good man sheweth favour, and lendeth: he will guide his affairs with discretion. He hath dispersed, he hath given to the poor; his righteousness endureth for ever; his horn shall be exalted with honour. (Psalm 112:5, 9)
- A man's pride shall bring him low: but honour shall uphold the humble in spirit. (Proverbs 29:23)

Way of healing
Confess that you have not been honouring and fearing God, that you have esteemed the things of God lightly, and that your life has become dishonourable. Acknowledge the Lordship of Christ and bow to His will. Then ask for your healing.

Helpful scriptures
Proverbs 3:13, 16

Mental illness, Alcoholism *(see also* <u>Depression</u>*)*

Spiritual cause: **idolatry**

Scriptures
- Babylon hath been a golden cup in the LORD's hand, that made all the earth drunken: the nations have drunken of her wine; therefore the nations are mad. (Jeremiah 51:7)
- I will do these things unto thee, because thou hast gone a whoring after the heathen, and because thou art polluted with their idols. Thou hast walked in the way of thy sister; therefore will I give her cup into thine hand. Thus saith the Lord GOD; Thou shalt drink of thy sister's cup deep and large: thou shalt be laughed to scorn and had in derision; it containeth much. Thou shalt be filled with drunkenness and sorrow, with the cup of astonishment and desolation, with the cup of thy sister Samaria. (Ezekiel 23:30-33)

- With whom the kings of the earth have committed fornication, and the inhabitants of the earth have been made drunk with the wine of her fornication. (Revelation 17:2)
- Jeremiah 13:10-13

Explanation of connection

The Bible describes the effect of idolatry upon an individual or a nation as drunkenness. As they follow after an idol, they show many of the effects of drunkenness: they lose their good sense and become mad; they are filled with a false feeling of wellbeing and happiness; they feel a compulsion to pursue it unceasingly; it leaves them in a state of ruin.

If we follow an idol of some kind, whether it be money, ambition, material possessions, relationships, academic prowess or fame, we will become drunk from it, losing our reason and ruining our lives. Ultimately we will be left with nothing.

Both mental illness and alcoholism/heavy drinking are a direct result of idolatry.

Mental illness

In practical terms, people's minds become ill when they follow after and are obsessed by something that is not God. Sometimes when a family member dies – a husband, wife, child or parent – an individual will spend all their time focussing on the one they have lost. They lose sight of God their creator and their late family member becomes the centre of their lives.

> Because that, when they knew God, they glorified him not as God, neither were thankful; but became vain in their imaginations, and their foolish heart was darkened. ...Who changed the truth of God into a lie, and worshipped and served the creature more than the Creator, who is blessed for ever. ... And even as they did not like to retain God in their knowledge, God gave them over to a reprobate mind. (Romans 1:21, 25, 28)

However, other things can become the focus of our obsessions: Christian service, some particular goal, spiritual or doctrinal perfection, a particular person, a well-known person, money or material possessions.

Way of healing
The idolatry needs to be understood and confessed. Anything that has taken central place in our lives and stopped God himself from being our focus must be confessed and forsaken. God desires to be our all in all, our source of happiness and fulfilment. Only He can satisfy our hearts.

Alcoholism and other addictions
All addictions are a form of idolatry. The person has made the thing that they are addicted to into a god: something upon which they rely and cannot live without. It is a crutch to help them get through life.

By confessing that they have made the thing into a god and being cleansed, they are delivered from the addiction.

When a person has an idolatrous nature, he will very often have numerous idols in his life: one form of idolatry quickly leads to another. Therefore, idolizing a person, for example, may lead to alcoholism. In order to get right with God and deal with one idol, we need to confess all areas of idolatry. Only then can God have His rightful place at the centre of our lives.

Helpful scriptures
Exodus 20:1-6; Joshua 24:1-28; Psalm 24; Hosea 2

Miscarriage

Spiritual cause: idolising one's children

Scriptures
- Thou shalt not bow down to their gods, nor serve them, nor do after their works: but thou shalt utterly overthrow them, and quite break down their images. And ye shall serve the LORD your God, and he shall bless thy bread, and thy

water; and I will take sickness away from the midst of thee. There shall nothing cast their young, nor be barren, in thy land: the number of thy days I will fulfil. (Exodus 23:24-26)

- Though they **bring up** their children, yet will I bereave them, that there shall not be a man left: yea, woe also to them when I depart from them! Ephraim, as I saw Tyrus, is planted in a pleasant place: but Ephraim shall bring forth his children to the murderer. Give them, O LORD: what wilt thou give? give them a miscarrying womb and dry breasts. (Hosea 9:12-14)

The Hebrew word for *bring up* is elsewhere translated *magnify* (Psalm 35:26; Isaiah 10:15; Daniel 11:36) to *boast* (Ezekiel 35:13) *advance* (Esther 10:2) *promote* (Esther 3:1) *speak proudly* (Obadiah 12).

Explanation of connection

When we have children, we can start to idolise them and make them our gods. We think about nothing but them, and speak about them all the time. They are the focus of our whole lives, our joy is bound up in them and they have taken the place of God.

God says that He hates idolatry. If we idolise our children and then start to have some more, he may allow the unborn child to die. This is to show us how we have departed from Him, and started worshipping our own children. Idolizing the unborn child may also cause a miscarriage (thus many people miscarry their first child).

How healing comes

Realise that children are a gift from God, but they should never take the place of God. God should be the centre of our whole lives – our joy, our happiness, our interest in life – and allowing anything to usurp that position is idolatry. Confess that you have made idols of your children and allow the Lord to cleanse you from this sin.

Helpful scriptures
Exodus 20:1-6; Luke 14:26; Psalm 142:5; Psalm 119:57;
The story of Mephibosheth and his relationship with David, a
type of Christ: II Samuel 9:1-13; II Samuel 19:24-39; II Samuel
16:1-4

Mouth

Spiritual meaning: relates to speech

Scriptures
- Let the words of my mouth, and the meditation of my heart, be acceptable in thy sight, O LORD, my strength, and my redeemer. (Psalm 19:14)

Explanation of connection
Since the mouth is the chief vehicle of speech, it is to be expected that when our mouths are affected by illness, it relates to our words. The biblical relationship between *words* and *the mouth* is clear: it is the mouth that does the speaking.

That which is gone out of thy lips thou shalt keep and perform; even a freewill offering, according as thou hast vowed unto the LORD thy God, which thou hast promised **with thy mouth.** (Deuteronomy 23:23)

Therefore, when our physical mouths become ill it symbolises the fact that we speak inappropriately.

Tongue, lips and other mouth problems
- Nevertheless they did flatter him with their mouth, and they lied unto him with their tongues. (Psalm 78:36)
- With persuasive words, she led him astray. With the flattering of her lips, she seduced him. (Proverbs 7:21)
- Their throat is an open sepulchre; with their tongues they have used deceit; the poison of asps is under their lips: whose mouth is full of cursing and bitterness. (Romans 3:13, 14)

The lips and tongue are used interchangeably as vehicles for inappropriate speech. The two things most frequently used in connection with the lips and tongue are lying and flattery, but any misuse of speech may bring a diseased mouth. These may include criticism, nagging, gossiping, insensitive or harsh speech, swearing and cursing, unkind words, boasting, being sharp-tongued, and speaking when you should remain silent. The biggest field for the misuse of speech is the home. This will often arise out of bad relationships: husbands not loving their wives, wives not submitting to their husbands, parents not loving their children and children not honouring their parents.

Our words have a huge effect; they may discourage or edify. Gossip is like a fire, starting very small but spreading until it has caused havoc and ruined lives.

> And the tongue is a fire, a world of iniquity: so is the tongue among our members, that it defileth the whole body, and setteth on fire the course of nature; and it is set on fire of hell. (James 3:6)

Our words also defile us if they are inappropriate (Matthew 15:11). They can also steer and influence our whole lives (James 3:3-4). James says,

> For in many things we offend all. If any man offend not in word, the same is a perfect man, and able also to bridle the whole body. (James 3:2)

For these reasons we need to learn to be careful in what we say, speaking out of love.

Way of Healing
Admit that you speak inappropriately. Seek to know just how you misuse your speech, and confess it before the Lord. Then ask for your healing.

Helpful scriptures
Ephesians 5; James 3

Saliva

Saliva is secreted into the mouth when food is taken, dissolving and lubricating certain foods and beginning the digestive process.

Since *water* symbolises *words,* saliva speaks of the words we say in conversation, our response which helps us to understand, enjoy and relate to people. When someone speaks, we reply and ask questions, enabling us to make the most of their words. An excess of saliva will indicate an excess of words in conversation; a dry mouth will indicate a shortage of words, such as failing to say enough to make oneself clear. A dry mouth can also lead to halitosis.

Cleft lip/palate *(see also* Congenital disorders*)*

This is a congenital disorder (a disorder from birth) and simply means that the lip or roof of the mouth is split open. It can be partial or complete. A complete cleft palate means there is a complete split from the lips to the back of the mouth. This means that the divide between the mouth and the nasal cavity is breached. This condition obviously impedes speech.

The nasal cavity and the mouth have connected but distinctly different roles. When we speak and eat, we also breathe through our noses at the same time (thus to speak with a blocked nose is most uncomfortable). Therefore the activities of the mouth (eating and speaking) need to happen simultaneously with the activities of the nose (breathing and smelling).

The mouth symbolises our exchange of words as we fellowship with other people *(See also* Digestive System, *page 148)*. When we speak we are feeding other people. When we take in other people's words, we are being fed.

> Man shall not live by bread alone, but by every word that proceedeth out of the mouth of God. (Matthew 4:4)

However, alongside our speaking and feeding, we should still have our continual relationship with God; we should still be *breathing* the Holy Spirit on a continual basis. This communion with God is distinct from but goes alongside the other activities. This enables us to perceive spiritually what is being said. (*See also* Smell). For each of the areas to function properly they need to be independent, even though they are connected.

When someone has a cleft palate, the mouth and nose become no longer separate. This means that the function of both is impaired. The nose cannot smell and clean the air adequately; the mouth cannot eat properly or speak properly. In spiritual terms, therefore, this symbolises someone who does not make a divide between their own spiritual existence and the words that they speak and receive. They have no independent, private spiritual faculty which is divorced from their relationship with people. In practice, when they speak, they will give everything away in their words, saying everything in their mind. When they listen, they will take things in very literally, without properly perceiving what they are, but then have difficulty coping with them.

The speech impediment that goes alongside it is an obvious indication of the fact that the person cannot clearly express himself, because of their inability to maintain a simultaneous private spiritual connection with God.

Way of healing
Confess that you do not maintain your own private spiritual life alongside but separate from your communication with people. Then ask for your healing.

Dumbness, Vocal problems

Spiritual cause: inappropriate use of the voice

Scriptures
- But I, as a deaf man, heard not; and I was as a dumb man that openeth not his mouth. Thus I was as a man that heareth not, and in whose mouth are no reproofs. (Psalm 38:13)
- And Zacharias said unto the angel, Whereby shall I know this? for I am an old man, and my wife well stricken in years.

And the angel answering said unto him, I am Gabriel, that stand in the presence of God; and am sent to speak unto thee, and to shew thee these glad tidings. And, behold, thou shalt be dumb, and not able to speak, until the day that these things shall be performed, because thou believest not my words, which shall be fulfilled in their season. (Luke 1:18-20)

- Now, brethren, if I come unto you speaking with tongues, what shall I profit you, except I shall speak to you either by revelation, or by knowledge, or by prophesying, or by doctrine? And even things without life giving sound, whether pipe or harp, except they give a distinction in the sounds, how shall it be known what is piped or harped? For if the trumpet give an uncertain sound, who shall prepare himself to the battle? So likewise ye, except ye utter by the tongue words easy to be understood, how shall it be known what is spoken? for ye shall speak into the air. (I Corinthians 14:6-9)

Explanation of connection

Our voice is what we use to express ourselves. It symbolises whether we are expressing what we ought to express.

We have been given our voices for a purpose: above all to praise God, but also to say things that ought to be said, to say things that are right and true and helpful and honest, things that honour God and things that come from God. When we use our voice inappropriately, we may lose it. This is a merciful provision of the Lord because it helps to prevent us saying things we will regret and that might cause damage.

When Zacharias uses his voice inappropriately, doubting the word of the messenger of God, he loses it for a time. Later on, however, he starts to walk with God again and regain his discernment. When asked what his newborn son should be called, he starts to express himself appropriately, giving the correct God-ordained name for the child. As a result, God enables him to speak and he goes on using his voice profitably by praising God.

And his mouth was opened immediately, and his tongue loosed, and he spake, and praised God. (Luke 1:64)

He lost his voice because he was not expressing what he ought to express. This was caused by unbelief.

Those who are filled with unbelief and therefore not filled with the Spirit will be unable to express themselves, to cry out to God and praise Him. Thus, in the case of a complete unbeliever, their dumbness is understandable: until they are born again they will not be able to express themselves and praise God.

Any misuse of the voice may bring vocal problems. This will include saying things that are foolish, unkind and inappropriate. It will be found that when, in the middle of speaking, a person starts to have difficulty with their voice, a frog in the throat or a cough, it is because they are starting to say something they shouldn't. Things said in the Spirit will often be given weight by a clear and powerful voice. Things said in the flesh will often be stifled by a weak voice. This is also true of singing: when, in an assembly, an appropriate hymn or song is chosen, it will be taken up and sung in good voice; equally, an inappropriate song, either because it is not right for the occasion or because it was not inspired by God, will be sung poorly and with difficulty.

There is also a link with another illness: <u>acid reflux</u>. Acid reflux can be caused by speaking of things from the past that should be forgotten. Acid reflux can also affect the voice. So this inappropriate use of the voice has two effects, one leading to the other.

Way of healing

The only way that we can speak the words that are pleasing to God, that are always appropriate, is to be filled with the spirit. In Ephesians 5 Paul condemns unprofitable speech, but then goes on to talk about how to say that which is profitable:

> Be filled with the Spirit; Speaking to yourselves in psalms and hymns and spiritual songs, singing and making melody in your heart to the Lord; giving thanks always for all things unto God and the Father in the name of our Lord Jesus Christ. (Ephesians 5:18-20)

Admit that you do not express yourself as you should. Be filled with the Spirit. This comes through getting right with God by confessing all known sin (and allowing Him to search you to reveal hidden sins) and allowing Him to control your life.

Helpful scriptures
Ephesians 5:1-21; James 3

Speech impediment
A speech impediment is something which prevents the normal flow of speech, such as a stutter. All speech impediments indicate that the person is stopping themselves expressing what they really ought, and perhaps want, to say. Just as physically their words are not able to come out, so in what they actually say they are not conveying the things they ought to say, the true reality of their hearts: they are not communicating straightforwardly. There may be various reasons for this, such as fear and nervousness, as well as pride. A person may be too afraid or too proud to say boldly and straightforwardly what they should say. This may be because they do not want to look foolish, are not willing to bend to the wishes of other people and say what would be right and helpful, or because they want to get their words absolutely correct (a kind of perfectionism).

We see this in Judges 12. The men of Ephraim are angry with Jephthah because he went into battle against the Ammonites without asking for their help. In fact, when Jephthah had asked for their help, they would not oblige, so he went into battle alone. When he was victorious, however, the men of Ephraim are jealous of his spoil. Consequently, when they threaten to burn down Jephthah's house on top of him, he fights against them and is victorious. When only a few of the Ephraimites are left and are trying to get across the Jordan, Jephthah's men, the Gileadites test them to see if they are Ephraimites.

And the Gileadites took the passages of Jordan before the Ephraimites: and it was so, that when those Ephraimites which were escaped said, Let me go over; that the men of Gilead said unto him, Art thou an Ephraimite? If he said, Nay; Then said they unto him, Say now Shibboleth: and he said Sibboleth: for he could not frame to pronounce it right. Then they took him, and slew him at the passages of Jordan. (Judges 12:5-6)

The Ephraimites were a selfish, proud and unfaithful people here. They were not careful with their words, failing to speak the truth to Jephthah. Thus when they are given the test of pronouncing the word *shibboleth* they fail to pronounce it correctly.

Stutter

A stutter is an impediment in which normal speech is interrupted or blocked by the repetition of parts of words and phrases, or by pauses. This indicates that a person is holding back from expressing themselves fully, from saying what they really mean. They have certain things they wish to say but they stop themselves from saying them, instead repeating things they have said before, saying things in part, or saying things they don't really want to say. This may be because of pride, or fear and nervousness.

Cluttering

Cluttering is when a person clutters up their sentences with endless explanations which hinder the true conveyance of the message. For example, instead of saying, 'I saw a dog bite a man today', a clutterer would say, 'Today, at some point, this morning I think, it may not have been a man – it could have been a woman – but I think it was a man, when I was in the park, I saw him being bitten by – well that's how it looked to me – a dog.'

When a person is worried or nervous about how their words are going to be received, they cease to focus on just conveying the important piece of information, focusing instead on the words they are actually saying and being distracted by other thoughts. They therefore add in explanations and other thoughts that enter the mind.

Way of healing

Recognise that you are not willing clearly and straightforwardly to express the things you ought to say. Confess this to God, humble yourself to speak boldly and plainly those things that are appropriate, and ask for your healing.

Halitosis (Bad Breath)

Spiritual cause: offensive speech

Scriptures
- Let no corrupt [putrid, rotten] communication proceed out of your mouth, but that which is good to the use of edifying, that it may minister grace unto the hearers. And grieve not the holy Spirit of God, whereby ye are sealed unto the day of redemption. Let all bitterness, and wrath, and anger, and clamour, and evil speaking, be put away from you, with all malice: And be ye kind one to another, tenderhearted, forgiving one another, even as God for Christ's sake hath forgiven you. (Ephesians 4:29-32)

Explanation of connection
When we say things to people that they don't want to hear, the Bible says it is like a bad smell. When, for example, Job spoke words that were offensive to his wife, his breath is described as strange to her:

My breath is strange to my wife, though I intreated for the children's sake of mine own body. (Job 19:17)

Similarly, we are told that, when we preach the gospel, it will come across as a foul smell to those that are perishing (who don't want to hear it), but to those that are saved (and appreciate the message), it is a pleasant fragrance:

For we are unto God a sweet savour of Christ, in them that are saved, and in them that perish: to the one we are the savour of death unto death; and to the other the savour of life unto life. (II Corinthians 2:15, 16)

God says that those who speak self-righteously are a stench in His nostrils, because their words are offensive to Him:

...Which say, Stand by thyself, come not near to me; for I am holier than thou. These are a smoke in my nose, a fire that burneth all the day. (Isaiah 65:5)

Therefore, when we suffer from bad breath, it is a demonstration that our words are offensive to those we speak to. We are not careful to ensure that what we are saying is going to be appreciated by the listener.

In conversation, for example, we may talk about the things that interest us, rather than saying things that are of mutual interest and of interest to the other person. We may have a hobby we like to talk about, or we may be obsessed with our work and talk about that to everyone. Just because these things are interesting to us, it doesn't mean that they are interesting to others. If our words are of no interest, they are like a foul smell to people.

Alternatively, we may simply be rude to people, especially those in our families. We may complain or criticise, or answer ungraciously. Equally we may say things that are coarse and unedifying.

Anything that is spoken that is insensitive and unwelcome to the listener may cause halitosis. Paul says to the Ephesians,

> Let no corrupt [putrid, rotten] communication proceed out of your mouth, but that which is good to the use of edifying, that it may minister grace unto the hearers. And grieve not the holy Spirit of God, whereby ye are sealed unto the day of redemption. Let all bitterness, and wrath, and anger, and clamour, and evil speaking, be put away from you, with all malice: and be ye kind one to another, tenderhearted, forgiving one another, even as God for Christ's sake hath forgiven you. (Ephesians 4:29-32)

The words here for *corrupt* and *mouth* when joined together form the Greek word for bad breath. Paul says, let your words not be foul to one another, but let them be spoken in love, to build people up. If we are truly loving, we will always want to say things that will be appreciated and do people good. Even when we have to correct people, if we say it lovingly, it can be received gladly (Ephesians 4:15).

Part of our living in a sacrificial way, laying down our lives for others, is speaking words in love. This then becomes a sweet savour.

And walk in love, as Christ also hath loved us, and hath given himself for us an offering and a sacrifice to God for a sweetsmelling savour. (Ephesians 5:2)

(In the case of the preaching of the gospel, obviously we preach it to everyone, but if we find people who adamantly do not want to hear, there is no point continuing to speak to them. This is casting pearls before swine.)

Way of healing
Admit that your words have often been unedifying to others, and not spoken out of regard for their feelings and situation. See that you need to be sensitive in what you say and think of the other person. Ask the Lord to cleanse you and then ask for your healing.

Muscle

Spiritual meaning: relates to strength

Scriptures
* Is my strength the strength of stones? or is my flesh of brass? (Job 6:12)

Explanation of connection
Inasmuch as the muscle is the part of a person's body which produces force and enables movement, in the spiritual it speaks of a person's spiritual force (that is, strength to act or move in spiritual things). A person with weak and wasting muscles has a lack of spiritual force.

Since our strength can only come from God, if we are weak spiritually it is because we have ceased to depend upon Him for our strength. Paul says to the Ephesians,

Finally, my brethren, be strong in the Lord, and in the power of his might. (Ephesians 6:10)

When the Psalmist says in Psalm 73 that his flesh fails, it comes after he has related that he had momentarily ceased to put his trust in the Lord. This very nearly causes him to fall.

My feet were almost gone; my steps had well nigh slipped. For I was envious at the foolish, when I saw the prosperity of the wicked. My flesh and my heart faileth: but God is the strength of my heart, and my portion for ever. (Psalm 73:2-3, 26)

The failure of his muscles causes him to put his trust back in the Lord, to find his strength in Him.

Diaphragm

The diaphragm is a muscular structure which separates the thorax (the cavity containing the heart and lungs) from the abdomen (containing the intestines, liver etc.). It is the main muscle used in breathing: by contracting it draws air into the lungs, by relaxing, the lungs are enabled to expel air. It is the muscle used in expelling things from the body: a foetus in childbirth, faeces and urine, and is active in vomiting, coughing, and sneezing.

In spiritual terms, this speaks of inner strength – resolve, decisiveness and integrity: strength for the internal spiritual life. In order to confess sins, in order to draw on the Holy Spirit, there needs to be a strength and resolve. It is not a passive action.

Hiccupping is the spasmodic contraction of the diaphragm which causes the sudden intake of air. This is an indication of a spasmodic attitude, often marked by foolish ideas and lack of steadiness.

Cramp

A cramp is a contraction (tightening) of a muscle. It indicates a restrictive attitude, a holding back. This may be in the leg or arm, indicating an unwillingness to move forward or to act, or in the bowels (*see* bowel cramp, *page 157).*

Way of healing

Confess that you haven't been depending upon God for your strength, but rather that you have depended upon yourself. See that your strength can be found in God alone.

Helpful scriptures

Psalm 27; II Corinthians 12:1-10

Neck

Spiritual meaning: relates to submission

Scriptures

- Judah, thou art he whom thy brethren shall praise: thy hand shall be in the neck of thine enemies; thy father's children shall bow down before thee. (Genesis 49:8)
- Therefore shalt thou serve thine enemies which the LORD shall send against thee, in hunger, and in thirst, and in nakedness, and in want of all things: and he shall put a yoke of iron upon thy neck, until he have destroyed thee. (Deuteronomy 28:48)
- For I know thy rebellion, and thy stiff neck: behold, while I am yet alive with you this day, ye have been rebellious against the LORD; and how much more after my death? (Deuteronomy 31:27)
- Greet Priscilla and Aquila my helpers in Christ Jesus: Who have for my life laid down their own necks: unto whom not only I give thanks, but also all the churches of the Gentiles. (Romans 16:3-4)

Explanation of connection

The neck is the part of an animal that bears the yoke. If an animal is determined to go its own way, it must stiffen its neck in order to pull the yoke in the direction in which it wants to go. To go in the right direction is easy – to resist the guidance of the yoke is hard work.

In spiritual terms, our yoke speaks of our submission to the Lord Jesus and to other people. The Lord Jesus says that as Christians we no longer need to worry. He has taken our sins upon Himself and He has promised to care for us in every way: therefore we can trust Him.

Come unto me, all ye that labour and are heavy laden, and I will give you rest. (Matthew 11:28)

All He now calls us to do is to obey Him. He tells us that the yoke He gives is easy:

> Take my yoke upon you, and learn of me; for I am meek and lowly in heart: and ye shall find rest unto your souls. For my yoke is easy, and my burden is light. (Matthew 11:29-30)

When we prefer to go our own way rather than Christ's, we are resisting His yoke. Our spiritual life becomes more difficult and we start to move out of His will. If physically we have a stiff neck, it means we have stiffened our neck spiritually.

Inasmuch as we are called to submit to one another and to those in authority over us (Ephesians 5:21), when we stiffen our necks and pull in our own direction against people our physical neck may be affected.

The Bible distinguishes between the yoke which Christ gives us and the yoke of legalism.

> Stand fast therefore in the liberty wherewith Christ hath made us free, and be not entangled again with the yoke of bondage. (Galatians 5:1; see also Acts 15:10)

When we take upon ourselves a yoke of slavery to the law rather than walking in the freedom that Christ has provided for us, it is an example of failing to walk in submission to Christ and we may suffer neck problems.

Way of healing

The Lord Jesus says that we should learn of Him and be meek and lowly – walking in obedience to God. We can be sure that God's way is best for us and that by submitting to Him and being obedient, we will be happiest.

Confess that you have resisted God's will. Be willing to submit to Him and obey Him, and then ask for your healing.

Helpful scriptures

I Peter 5:5-7

Neurological

Spiritual meaning: **use of mind**

Scriptures
- For they that are after the flesh do mind the things of the flesh; but they that are after the Spirit the things of the Spirit. For to be carnally minded is death; but to be spiritually minded is life and peace. Because the carnal mind is enmity against God: for it is not subject to the law of God, neither indeed can be. (Romans 8:5-7)

Explanation of connection
As might be expected, the brain and nervous system represents the mind and the way in which we use our mind to control areas of our lives.

Cerebral palsy
- LORD, I know that the way of man is not in himself: it is not in man that walketh to direct his steps. (Jeremiah 10:23)
- The steps of a good man are ordered by the LORD: and he delighteth in his way. Though he fall, he shall not be utterly cast down: for the LORD upholdeth him with his hand. (Psalm 37:23-24)

Cerebral palsy covers a range of conditions in which movement of the body is impaired through damage to the brain or a failure in its development. As this occurs in infancy or in the womb, this will indicate certain problems in the lives of the parents that, without intervention, the child is bound to repeat (see What about children?, page 53). In particular, it will mean that different areas of a person's life, especially his actions, are not being controlled. This may mean either that they are not being controlled at all, or it may mean that our lives are controlled without wisdom.

The Bible says that our steps should be ordered by the Lord. If we allow the Lord to control us, we can be sure that our actions are wisely directed.

How healing comes

Confess that your steps have been directed without wisdom, and see that they need to be ordered. Ask the Lord to order them and ask for your healing/the healing of your child

Stroke

A stroke occurs when the supply of blood to part of the brain is interrupted. Some brain cells start to die and others become damaged.

In the spiritual, this speaks of when a mind is not consecrated to God. Deuteronomy 12:23 says that 'the blood is the life'. Just as our body sends blood to the brain for it to operate properly, in order for our mind to work well, it needs to be supplied by life. This means being given over to God – enlivened by him, used in His strength and used for something good and worthwhile. When we are particularly gifted mentally, we can become proud. This can mean that we start to depend on our own mental ability, even in Christian work, rather than depending upon God. It can also mean that we put it to uses which we think are worthwhile but which are not of God. Obviously, the things that are useful are those that the Holy Spirit wants us to be involved in, the spiritual life:

> I beseech you therefore, brethren, by the mercies of God, that ye present your bodies a living sacrifice, holy, acceptable unto God, which is your reasonable service. And be not conformed to this world: but **be ye transformed by the renewing of your mind**, that ye may prove what is that good, and acceptable, and perfect, will of God. For I say, through the grace given unto me, to every man that is among you, not to think of himself more highly than he ought to think; but to think soberly, according as God hath dealt to every man the measure of faith. (Romans 12:1-3)

When we have a stroke, it forces us to depend upon God for our mental ability rather than depending upon ourselves.

How healing comes

We may have been blessed with a very good brain of which we're proud, but we may have been putting it to worldly use, or tried to use it in our own strength. Unless our mind is given over to God to be used for His purposes, it is of no spiritual eternal value. Confess that you have not given your mind over to the things of God to be used by Him.

Helpful Scriptures

Romans 8:5-7; Daniel 4:28-37

Parkinson's disease

Parkinson's disease involves the loss of brain cells in the part of the brain responsible for movement. The main symptoms are tremor, stiffness, lack of balance in walking and other difficulties in movement.

In spiritual terms, Parkinson's speaks of someone who has ceased to move forward. For various reasons, such as fear, complacency or lack of spiritual interest, the person has stopped going on with God into new spiritual territory.

The children of Israel experienced this spiritual state as recorded in Exodus 14. After escaping from Egypt and as they approach the Red Sea, they looked back to see Pharaoh pursuing, 'and they were sore afraid' (Exodus 14:10). Their reaction was to desire to return to Egypt.

In response to this, the Lord told Moses that their mistake was in failing to move forward.

> And the LORD said unto Moses, Wherefore criest thou unto me? speak unto the children of Israel, that they go forward. (Exodus 14:15)

The children of Israel needed to go forward, trusting the Lord, in order to reach finally the promised land.

The same principle is evident in the parable of the talents in Matthew 25:14-30. The servant who was given one talent buried it out of fear of making a mistake. His master is furious with him for being unprofitable.

Parkinson's disease will often come on people who have gone far with God but then stopped.

Way of healing
Perhaps out of fear of making a mistake, or perhaps out of complacency, laziness, inertia or too much interest in the things of the world, you have failed to continue moving forward in your Christian life. See that the Lord has unbounded blessings to those who continue to go forward with Him. Confess that your Christian life has become stagnant, express your desire to go on with God, and then ask for your healing.

Helpful scriptures
I Corinthians 2:9;

Epilepsy

Spiritual cause: the pride of life, intellectual pride

Scriptures
- Daniel 4:28-37
- …those that walk in pride he is able to abase. (Daniel 4:37b)
- Let him that thinketh he standeth take heed lest he fall. (I Corinthians 10:12)

Explanation of connection
There is a particular failing which the Bible describes as 'the pride of life' (I John 2:16). This is a pride in our very existence, a pride in who we are and what we can do. We may, for example, feel we are very gifted intellectually or physically, or we may be proud of our success. We may think that our gifts are of our own making. In response to this, God may humble us.

Epilepsy strikes at the centre of this problem. During a seizure, the normal operations of the brain are utterly disrupted and we become more helpless than a baby: we are completely unable to control ourselves. We are instantly forced into a place of deep humility, to admit that, without the grace of God, we are utterly incapable of anything.

In the book of Daniel, Nebuchadnezzar is lifted up with pride. He says,

Is not this great Babylon, that I have built for the house of the kingdom by the might of my power, and for the honour of my majesty? (Daniel 4:28)

In response, God allows him to become ill with a disease that, like epilepsy, deeply humbles him.

The same hour was the thing fulfilled upon Nebuchadnezzar: and he was driven from men, and did eat grass as oxen, and his body was wet with the dew of heaven, till his hairs were grown like eagles' feathers, and his nails like birds' claws. (Daniel 4:33)

The illness does its work, and Nebuchadnezzar returns to his senses.

And at the end of the days I Nebuchadnezzar lifted up mine eyes unto heaven, and mine understanding returned unto me, and I blessed the most High, and I praised and honoured him that liveth for ever, whose dominion is an everlasting dominion, and his kingdom is from generation to generation. (Daniel 4:34)

The way of healing
Confess that you have been proud of who you are and what you can do, that you have thought that your abilities were of your own making rather than only existing by the grace of God; confess that without God's upholding power you can do nothing, and that He alone is worthy of honour and praise.

Helpful scriptures
I Corinthians 4:7; I Peter 5:5; Psalm 29:1, 2

Encephalitis
Encephalitis is an inflammation of the brain. This indicates that our mind is not being used as it should, that it has become

damaged in some way, infected by sin; there is a problem in the way we think. This may result from various causes.

Naturally, the human mind is impaired. It therefore needs to be renewed.

And be not conformed to this world: but be ye transformed by the renewing of your mind, that ye may prove what is that good, and acceptable, and perfect, will of God. (Romans 12:2)

When our mind is conformed to the world, it is diseased, it does those things which are inappropriate, it seeks to please us rather than God. However, if we come to God and ask Him to give us the mind of Christ, to think as He would have us think, then our mind is renewed and restored.

How healing comes
Confess that your mind has not been conformed to Christ's, that it has been adversely influenced, such as by the world. Ask Him to give you His mind so that your mind may be guided and used by Him to do His work. Ask for your healing.

Meningitis
The *meninges* are the membranes that enclose and protect the central nervous system – the brain and the spinal chord. When they become diseased, it is an indication that we are not showing respect and regard to our mind, perhaps abusing it by overloading it, using it for worthless things, and not giving it freedom to work. Sometimes we may be impatient and try and drive our minds too hard.

Hydrocephalus
The brain produces a liquid called cerebrospinal fluid which normally passes into the cavity surrounding the brain where it helps to protect the brain by forming a cushion. It then flows down the spinal chord before being released into the veins. With hydrocephalus, the fluid that is produced fails to drain away from the head, causing pressure to build up within the skull.

Since *water* represents *words,* the cerebrospinal fluid represents the words, or intelligent output, produced by the mind. The use of our minds in intelligent reasoning helps to protect them. This intelligence should then pass on and be put into action, and then be swept away as our lives move on.

In practical terms, a person's mind thinks various intelligent thoughts. These should then be put into effect, be used for something. They then become the thing of yesterday's life, as something new comes along.

If someone has intelligent thoughts, but never puts them into practice, never uses them for anything worthwhile, but simply retains them as intelligent thoughts, they are putting excessive pressure on their minds, as the intelligent words build up. When a person has hydrocephalus it is an indication of this.

Motor Neurone Disease

Motor neurones are the cells that control muscle activity in the body. When they are diseased, an individual loses the ability to control different parts of the body. These have an impact on many of the normal functions of life, including speech, movement and breathing.

This speaks of failing to control different areas of our spiritual lives. We may not control our thoughts, our words, or our actions. We may allow our minds to wander foolishly, saying things without thinking, and acting irrationally.

Alzheimer's

Alzheimer's disease involves the degeneration of neurones in the brain, causing deterioration in thinking processes. The most notable initial feature is loss of short term memory.

In spiritual terms this indicates spiritual forgetfulness: not remembering who God is, failing to remember what He has done, and consequently not being thankful.

For the invisible things of him from the creation of the world are clearly seen, being understood by the things that are made, even his eternal power and Godhead; so that they are without excuse: because that, when they knew God, they glorified him not as God, neither were thankful; but became vain in their imaginations, and their foolish heart was darkened. ...and even as they did not like to retain God in their knowledge, God gave them over to a reprobate mind, to do those things which are not convenient. (Romans 1:20-21, 28)

Alzheimer's serves to cause the sufferer to forget everything else so that they might remember God.

Way of healing
The individual needs to bring God back into their consciousness, as their creator and the giver of life. They need to recall who He is and what He has done for them. Confess the failing and ask for healing.

Multiple sclerosis
Multiple sclerosis is a disease in which the neurons (information-carrying cells of the brain and spinal chord) are damaged. Neurons are protected and aided by sheaths made of *myelin*, a substance consisting mainly of fat. Sometimes a person's own immune system starts attacking these sheaths and destroying them. The neurons themselves can also then be cut through.

Since *fat* speaks of our enjoyment (*see* Quick Reference), myelin speaks of the enjoyment that protects and insulates our minds and our decisions to act. When we enjoy life and enjoy the things that we do, this enables our minds and feelings to function well. However, sometimes our consciences may be over-sensitive, and we may worry about everything we do and say, wondering whether we should be doing it. Thus our enjoyment is destroyed and our ability to put into operation what our minds have determined is impaired.

It is interesting to note that one of the effects of multiple sclerosis is to give the individual affected a feeling of euphoria. This means that the person is forced to enjoy life, thus reversing the person's natural disposition.

Way of healing

Confess that you have become so nervous about doing things that it has stopped you enjoying life and so impaired your ability to put into effect what you have planned and decided to do. See that you can enjoy life, and trust the Lord to guide you.

Helpful Scriptures

Proverbs 17:22; I Timothy 6:17

Obesity, weight problems

Spiritual cause: big self life

Scriptures

- But Jeshurun waxed fat, and kicked: thou art waxen fat, thou art grown thick, thou art covered with fatness; then he forsook God which made him, and lightly esteemed the Rock of his salvation. (Deuteronomy 32:15)
- They are inclosed in their own fat: with their mouth they speak proudly. (Psalm 17:10)
- As a cage is full of birds, so are their houses full of deceit: therefore they are become great, and waxen rich. They are waxen fat, they shine: (Jeremiah 5:27, 28)

Explanation of connection

In scripture, our flesh stands for our humanity (e.g. Matthew 16:17). It is the natural man. Sometimes a person becomes very big in his own eyes. He sees himself as very important, he is always thinking about himself. The Bible describes this as growing fat.

> The proud have forged a lie against me: but I will keep thy precepts with my whole heart. Their heart is as fat as grease; but I delight in thy law. (Psalm 119:69-70)

Weight problems and obesity are the indication that someone has a big self-image. They feed their ego, they build themselves up.

Curiously, there are some emotions that go together with this that some may find surprising. A person may be shy, may feel very inadequate, may say they hate themselves, and yet have a big *self-life*. In actual fact these emotions are to be expected. Someone who cares and thinks a lot about themselves will inevitably be self-conscious. They want themselves to excel at everything, but when they find they fail, they are discouraged. When they say they hate themselves, they really mean that they love themselves and wish they were more gifted, better looking, more successful.

A big self-image does not mean that a person likes what they see in themselves, but that they spend a lot of time looking.

Way of Healing

The way to cease to be big in one's own eyes is to see ourselves as having been crucified with Christ. There is nothing good in our human nature: it is utterly corrupt. Paul says,

> For I know that in me (that is, in my flesh,) dwelleth no good thing: for to will is present with me; but how to perform that which is good I find not. For the good that I would I do not: but the evil which I would not, that I do. (Romans 7:18, 19)

Therefore, the old nature had to die. So when Christ died on the cross, we died with Him (Romans 6:6), so that our corrupt nature could be replaced by His victorious life.

> I am crucified with Christ: neverthless I live; yet not I, but Christ liveth in me: and the life which I now live in the flesh I live by the faith of the Son of God, who loved me, and gave himself for me. (Galatians 2:20)

Therefore, we should live as if our fleshly old nature is dead. That means putting to death everything that is to do with self: self interest, self-concern, self-pity, self-love, self-esteem. John the Baptist said of Christ, 'He must increase, but I must decrease' (John 3:30).

Tozer says,

> The victorious Christian neither exalts nor downgrades himself. His interests have shifted from self to Christ. What he is or is not

no longer concerns him. He believes that he has been crucified with Christ and he is not willing either to praise or deprecate such a man.[28]

Our focus, therefore, should be on the Lord and upon other people.

Let us run with patience the race that is set before us, looking unto Jesus the author and finisher of our faith (Hebrews 12:1-2) Let nothing be done through strife or vainglory; but in lowliness of mind let each esteem other better than themselves. Look not every man on his own things, but every man also on the things of others. (Philippians 2:4-5)

Helpful scriptures
Philippians 2:1-11

Parasite

Spiritual cause: **a parasite in one's life**

Scriptures
- Ye are not straitened in us, but ye are straitened in your own bowels. (II Corinthians 6:12)
- Behold, the third time I am ready to come to you; and I will not be burdensome to you: for I seek not yours but you: for the children ought not to lay up for the parents, but the parents for the children. And I will very gladly spend and be spent for you; though the more abundantly I love you, the less I be loved. But be it so, I did not burden you: nevertheless, being crafty, I caught you with guile. Did I make a gain of you by any of them whom I sent unto you? (II Corinthians 12:14-17)
- Let the elders that rule well be counted worthy of double honour, especially they who labour in the word and doctrine. For the scripture saith, Thou shalt not muzzle the ox that

---

[28] *Man – The Dwelling Place of God*, A. W. Tozer, Ch.18.

treadeth out the corn. And, The labourer is worthy of his
reward. (I Timothy 5:17-18)

Explanation of connection

A parasite is something that lives in our bodies or on them, and
which gets its nourishment from our bodies. Examples are the
malarial parasite, roundworms and tapeworms.

In spiritual terms, this speaks of people who are inappropriately
relying on us for their physical or spiritual provision. Some people
are in a position of real need and it is right to provide for them,
others may take advantage of our generosity, not pulling their
weight, and becoming a burden.

In I Timothy 5, Paul talks about several different cases of
providing for other people. In speaking about widows, he talks
about those who are real widows and those who are not. He says a
widow who is truly desolate, seemingly with no-one to look after
her, should be provided for by the church. However, those that
have families should be provided for by their families.

> Honour widows that are widows indeed. But if any widow have
> children or nephews, let them learn first to shew piety at home,
> and to requite their parents: for that is good and acceptable
> before God. If any man or woman that believeth have widows,
> let them relieve them, and let not the church be charged; that it
> may relieve them that are widows indeed. (I Timothy 5:3-4, 16)

Similarly, he says that elders who provide teaching within the
assembly should receive payment. In this way neither is being a
parasite: the elder is giving something to the church and the church
is giving something to the elder.

When we are inappropriately burdened by other people, we
become weak and sick. We see this in the case of Epaphroditus,
who was compelled to carry the burden that the Philippian church
should have borne.

> Because for the work of Christ he was nigh unto death, not
> regarding his life, to supply your lack of service toward me.
> (Philippians 2:27)

We need to discern between burdens that are right for us to carry and those that are not, and see that other people should do what is required of them in the Lord.

Way of healing
Confess that you have been taken advantage of and have not ensured that your relationship is two-way. See the lack of wisdom in this arrangement, and ask the Lord to remedy it.

Helpful scriptures
I Corinthians 9:1-14

Reproductive system, Male

Impotence
- Likewise, ye husbands, dwell with them according to knowledge, giving honour unto the wife, as unto the weaker vessel, and as being heirs together of the grace of life; that your prayers be not hindered. (I Peter 3:7)

Inasmuch as the man is said to be the stronger of the two and that the woman is to be in submission to him (Colossians 3:18), a man who is in submission to his wife, who has become weaker than she, has lost his rightful role. Impotence signifies this.

Prostate
- Let the husband render unto the wife due benevolence: and likewise also the wife unto the husband. The wife hath not power of her own body, but the husband: and likewise also the husband hath not power of his own body, but the wife. Defraud ye not one the other, except it be with consent for a time, that ye may give yourselves to fasting and prayer; and come together again, that Satan tempt you not for your incontinency. (I Corinthians 7:3-5)

Explanation of connection

The prostate gland is part of the male reproductive system that creates warmth of feeling towards the female sex. A diseased prostate gland indicates a lack of kindness and warm-heartedness towards women, whether it be a wife or any other woman.

Testicular diseases

- And thou shalt not let any of thy seed pass through the fire to Molech. (Leviticus 18:22)

The seed of a man speaks of two things: his children, and of seeds of things that a man produces, such as a plan, scheme or idea. Therefore, when the testicles are diseased, it indicates that the man has a wrong attitude towards his children or towards something else to which he has given birth, or is going to give birth.

a) Children

A diseased testicle may indicate a bad attitude towards children. This may include a lack of care for children, especially one's own, but also of any that you have an effect upon and for subsequent generations. A lack of diligent Christian service which causes subsequent generations to suffer could be seen as a lack of care for children:

One generation shall praise thy works to another, and shall declare thy mighty acts. (Psalm 145:4, *see also* Joshua 4)

Caring for children includes providing for them, disciplining them, ensuring that they thrive, protecting them from harm, ensuring that they grow up in the Lord:

And, ye fathers, provoke not your children to wrath: but bring them up in the nurture and admonition of the Lord. (Ephesians 6:4)

Causing or allowing one's wife to have an abortion is an example of letting your 'seed pass through the fire'. Failing to beget the children allotted to you (through contraception, vasectomy etc.) will also show a lack of love towards your children.

Undescended testes (*cryptorchidism*) indicate a disposition which means the individual will take a long time before God deems them ready to have children.

b) Plans

If you are thinking out a plan or idea, and there is something wrong in this process, it may be indicated by diseased testicles. The scheme itself may be wrong in itself – of the flesh or sinful, or perhaps God has given you an idea that you are thinking through and you have a bad attitude towards it – you don't want to carry it out.

Varicocele

In this condition the veins that drain blood away from the testicles can become swollen because the blood is not draining away properly. This indicates that the man is concentrating too much of his life on either his children or a plan that he has.

Way of healing

Confess the particular wrong attitude that you have and ask for your healing.

Helpful scriptures

Joshua 4; II Corinthians 12:14

Venerial diseases (*see also* HIV/AIDS)

- What? know ye not that he which is joined to an harlot is one body? for two, saith he, shall be one flesh. Flee fornication. Every sin that a man doeth is without the body; but he that committeth fornication sinneth against his own body. (I Corinthians 6:16, 18)
- Wherefore come out from among them, and be ye separate, saith the Lord, and touch not the unclean thing; and I will receive you. (II Corinthians 6:17)

These are related to sexual promiscuity. When a person joins themselves to someone in sexual activity which is outside a heterosexual marriage, they are joining themselves with uncleanness. This will have a number of results and symptoms.

The effects of venereal diseases on the skin indicate the uncleanness of the association within a sexual relationship (*see also* Skin). Bacterial and viral infections speak of the sin involved. Impotence indicates how the promiscuity has caused a man to become subject to women. Sores indicate a lack of care and concern about how a person is abusing their own life in this area. (Other symptoms, such as cold-like symptoms, may be seen under their own category).

Way of healing
In all cases of venereal diseases, the sexual promiscuity should be seen as gross uncleanness and confessed to God. When it is confessed and forsaken, He cleanses us from all the unrighteousness and gives us a clean heart and mind. Then full healing can come.

Helpful scriptures
II Samuel 11:1-12:23; Psalm 51, I John 1

Reproductive system, Female

Uterus
- The wicked man travaileth with pain all his days, and the number of years is hidden to the oppressor. (Job 15:
- For the congregation of hypocrites shall be desolate, and fire shall consume the tabernacles of bribery. They conceive mischief, and bring forth vanity, and their belly [womb] prepareth deceit. (Job 15:35)

After a child is conceived in the uterine tube, the uterus (or womb) is the place where a child is nourished and protected. It is the uterus that then expels the child when a woman gives birth.

In spiritual terms, this speaks of a woman's role in conceiving, nourishing and launching things out into the world. Primarily this speaks of a woman's children, but it may also speak of other things she produces. An action begins life as an idea, it is then nourished and becomes a plan, and finally it is brought forth. A diseased uterus is an indication that there is something wrong in the way she prepares things for being launched.

This may mean she is bringing up her children in a way that is wrong, or that she is not preparing them for life. Perhaps she is unwilling to have children or has a bad attitude towards her role in bringing them up.

Alternatively, it may speak of a problem in the way a woman plans things. This could mean that she devises plans that are not of God. This might range from plans that are simply pointless and fleshly, through to plans to harm other people. In many cases, a woman will have no intention of carrying out the plan, but may enjoy thinking about things she would like to do.

(See also Venereal diseases *under* Reproductive System, Male.)

Helpful scriptures
I Timothy 5:10; II Samuel 11:1-12:23; Psalm 51, I John 1

Respiratory *(for* Blood, *see under separate heading)*

Spiritual cause: relates to being spiritual/filled with the Holy Spirit

Scriptures
- And the LORD God formed man of the dust of the ground, and breathed into his nostrils the breath of life; and man became a living soul. (Genesis 2:7)
- Thus saith the Lord GOD unto these bones; Behold, I will cause breath to enter into you, and ye shall live. (Ezekiel 37:5)
- And when he had said this, he breathed on them, and saith unto them, Receive ye the Holy Ghost. (John 20:22)
- See then that ye walk circumspectly, not as fools, but as wise, redeeming the time, because the days are evil. Wherefore be ye not unwise, but understanding what the will of the Lord is. And be not drunk with wine, wherein is excess; but be filled with the Spirit; speaking to yourselves in psalms and hymns and spiritual songs, singing and making melody in your heart to the Lord; giving thanks always for all things unto God and the Father in the name of our Lord Jesus Christ; submitting yourselves one to another in the fear of God. (Ephesians 5:15-21)

Explanation of connection

When we breathe physically, the oxygen we need for life enters our bodies via our lungs and is carried round the body in the blood.

When God created man, He breathed life into his nostrils, making him a living soul. The air that he breathed represented the life of God entering him. Similarly, after the resurrection, when the Lord gave the disciples the Holy Spirit, it says that He breathed upon them.

As Christians, we need to breathe the Holy Spirit on a continual basis. The Bible describes this as *walking* in the spirit. It is like walking in fresh air, and breathing it in. It means being spiritual rather than carnal.

Romans 8 covers the subject in depth and shows the difference between walking in the Spirit (being spiritually minded) and walking in the flesh (being carnally minded). Walking in the Spirit means walking in continual fellowship with God: being guided by God, living in God's strength, seeing things as God sees them and doing everything for God's glory. Walking in the flesh is the opposite: being guided by our human instincts and desires, living in our own strength, seeing things in human terms, and doing them for our own glory and benefit. Paul says,

> For they that are after the flesh do mind the things of the flesh; but they that are after the Spirit the things of the Spirit. For to be carnally minded is death; but to be spiritually minded is life and peace. Because the carnal mind is enmity against God: for it is not subject to the law of God, neither indeed can be. So then they that are in the flesh cannot please God. But ye are not in the flesh, but in the Spirit, if so be that the Spirit of God dwell in you. Now if any man have not the Spirit of Christ, he is none of his. (Romans 8:5-9)

Walking in the flesh can include:

- Everything done in one's own strength rather than in God's, including prayer, Christian service, and living the Christian life
- Fleshly desires, such as lusts, ambition, greed, avarice

- Thinking about oneself, self-promotion, self-consciousness

When we have breathing difficulties, it means we are being unspiritual: we are not walking in the spirit but in the flesh. The causes of this can vary slightly, as seen in different types of breathing problems.

Nose

Since the nose is the route by which air is supposed to enter our bodies, difficulty breathing through the nose will mean lack of openness to the Holy Spirit and to the spiritual realm: we are not being spiritual at all. This may result from having so many things in our minds that we do not allow the Holy Spirit simply to move in us and have perfect access and control. It may be because we have lost our spiritual focus and need to get back in tune with the Holy Spirit. In all cases it is fundamentally due to fleshliness.

> Now if any man have not the Spirit of Christ, he is none of his [the Spirit's]. (Romans 8:9)

Lungs, including Asthma

After air has entered the body through the nose, it enters the blood through the lungs. In spiritual terms, this speaks of our response to the working of the Holy Spirit and the access we give Him into the depths of our lives. Very often our lives fill up with other things so that we limit the work of the Holy Spirit within us. These things especially include fleshly thoughts and words, which is symbolised by fluid in the lungs.

When someone has **asthma**, the airways within the lungs become inflamed and constrict (tighten and close up), limiting breathing. This is often triggered by factors such as allergens and viruses. In the spiritual this speaks of someone who allows the Holy Spirit into their life but is continually fighting Him. They hear Him guiding them, but are in contention, not fully letting Him have His way but nevertheless wanting to keep hearing from Him.

For the flesh lusteth against the Spirit, and the Spirit against the flesh: and these are contrary the one to the other: so that ye cannot do the things that ye would. (Galatians 5:17)

Colds and fevers (*see also* Infectious Diseases)

There are times in our lives when we over-estimate our own importance and believe that almost everything depends upon us. We may get rather overheated with work and with life, becoming like a machine that is overheated and spinning too fast. We get carried away with things, become excessively zealous, losing our calm, our sense of balance and our reason. Usually we are unaware that we are in this condition. As a result of this, we start to work and live in the flesh rather than in the spirit. We work in our own strength, for our own glory. Two things characterize this condition. First is the state of frenzy, in which we feel our own importance. We may be led to race round, being very active. The second is the fact that we are actually achieving hardly anything, because we are not being guided by God. Our fleshliness then causes us to sin: we have sinful attitudes and thoughts of which we are unaware, especially bad attitudes towards other people (see Infectious diseases). At this point we may get a cold.

All this is very much a product of pride, as we think that our work and our lives are so important. Thus God has to guide us back to the place where we should be.

When we become head-strong and unruly, we put ourselves in the position of Sennacherib, King of Assyria. In Isaiah, we read how God uses Sennacherib to chasten the Kingdom of Judah, though Sennacherib does not realise the beneficial role he is undertaking in coming against Judah (Isaiah 10:5-13). Sennacherib, however, responds to the situation with pride, believing that his power against Judah is of his own making. Therefore, God says to him:

Because thy rage against me, and thy tumult, is come up into mine ears, therefore will I put my hook in thy nose, and my bridle in thy lips, and I will turn thee back by the way by which thou camest. (Isaiah 37:29)

The word here for *tumult* literally means *to be at ease (to the point of arrogance),* so Sennacherib is described as both raging and arrogantly at ease.

When we get a cold, it is like having a hook put in our nose, to guide us back into the right way and to steer us with a firm hand when we have started to walk in the flesh. It acts very effectively in killing our fleshly attitudes. We have to slow down and refocus.

A fever indicates that we are in a fever spiritually – raging and overheated.

Way of healing

When we became Christians, the fleshly way of living, the 'old nature' was pronounced dead, so that we should walk in newness of life, that is, live by the spirit.

> And if Christ be in you, the body is dead because of sin; but the Spirit is life because of righteousness. (Romans 8:10).

However, as Christians, we sometimes let the old fleshly nature live. Paul says that we should put it to death.

> For if ye live after the flesh, ye shall die: but if ye through the Spirit do mortify the deeds of the body, ye shall live. (Romans 8:13)

Living in the Spirit means being guided by God, working in His strength and doing it for His glory. Living in the flesh means the opposite.

See that you have been living in the flesh, rather than in the Spirit, that you have been doing things in your own strength and for your own sake, rather than being dead to sin and self, and alive to God.

Helpful scriptures

Romans 7 & 8

Post nasal drip (PND)

- A continual dropping in a very rainy day and a contentious woman are alike. (Proverbs 27:15)

Post nasal drip is when mucus continues to drip from behind the nose down the throat. When we are contentious, our argumentative thoughts drip away all the time, and this comes out in our words: we may keep on and on, never giving anyone peace. PND is caused by the general flow of thoughts when we 'talk' in our minds, which is often a symptom of a contentious attitude. However, any flow of words in our minds may cause PND.

Just as PND limits our breathing, so the spiritual cause limits our walking in the spirit. PND can also clog up the tonsils, leading to tonsil infections and halitosis (see each of these under separate headings).

Contentiousness is always caused by pride:

Only by pride cometh contention: but with the well advised is wisdom. (Proverbs 13:10)

By confessing one's pride and being cleansed, healing can come.

Pleural cavity

The pleurae are the two membranes that surround the lungs, one inside the other. Their role is to help protect the lungs and enable their smooth functioning. They slide against each other as we inhale and exhale. The pleural cavity is the potential space that lies between the pleurae, which is wet with pleural fluid. This normally has negative pressure (like a vacuum). This means that the outer lining of the lungs is pulled outwards thus keeping them open.

In spiritual terms, the pleurae and pleural cavity speak of the things that surround our spiritual life, the things necessary to enable us to be filled with the Spirit. Chief amongst these is spiritual desire, an interest in spiritual things. Just as there is a negative pressure in the pleural cavity keeping the lungs open, there should be a certain *feeling of lack* that keeps us desiring spiritual things, keeps us open spiritually. In order to maintain this, it is important that we deprive ourselves of the things of the world. This makes it easier for us to be filled with the Holy Spirit when we come to God, because we have a longing, a desire to be filled. It makes us hungry for God:

Blessed are they which do hunger and thirst after righteousness: for they shall be filled. (Matthew 5:6)

When the negative pressure is not maintained in the pleural cavity, the lung collapses. This speaks of losing a desire for spiritual things. The lung may also collapse when the pleurae are punctured. This symbolises the fact that the Enemy has managed to wound us. He is always trying to attack us spiritually: when we sin or do something in the flesh, he is able to score a hit and wound us. This leaves us discouraged and deflated. We feel like giving up. The spiritual desire and tension that would naturally cause us to want to be filled with the Spirit has been lost.

Sometimes the pleural cavity fills with fluid, crushing the lung. Since *water* symbolises *words*, this speaks of when our spiritual life is so surrounded by *talk* that we don't have room to breathe: there isn't space to be filled with the Spirit.

Way of healing
Confess that you have lost your spiritual desire. Search your heart and ask the Holy Spirit to reveal the thing that led to the discouragement. It may be a sin, a mistake, an act of the flesh; it may be because you have filled your life with other things rather than God. Confess that sin to God and ask for your healing.

Pleurisy
Pleurisy is the inflammation of the pleurae: they become painful and uncomfortable, often as a result of infection. This speaks of a problem in our attitude towards spiritual things, especially the positive things that surround our spiritual lives (such as our church, personal devotions etc.). Our interest in the things of God may be contaminated because there is sin in our lives. There may be wrong motives in our spiritual desire. This stops us enjoying spiritual things. It means that our spiritual experience is painful and uncomfortable.

Way of healing
Confess that there is a problem with your spiritual desire, that there are things that have contaminated your walk with God and made it uncomfortable. Search your heart to know what these sins are and confess them one by one as they come to

mind. When you have confessed and forsaken every sin that you recognize in your life, ask for your healing.

Senses: taste, smell, feel

Spiritual meaning: relates to certain spiritual faculties

Taste – discernment

Scriptures
- Is there iniquity in my tongue? cannot my taste discern perverse things? (Job 6:30)
- I am this day fourscore years old: and can I discern between good and evil? can thy servant taste what I eat or what I drink? can I hear any more the voice of singing men and singing women? (II Samuel 19:35)
- Doth not the ear try words? and the mouth taste his meat? (Job 12:11)
- If so be ye have tasted that the Lord is gracious. (I Peter 2:3)

Explanation of connection
The food we eat speaks of our fellowship with God and with other people. When we taste something, we discern what it is we are eating. In the same way, in spiritual fellowship, we should exercise discernment, distinguishing between good and evil, carefully observing the true nature of the fellowship we are enjoying. It is said of the Lord Jesus,

> Butter and honey shall he eat, that he may know to refuse the evil, and choose the good. (Isaiah 7:15)

When we have lost our sense of taste, it means that we are no longer exercising our discernment in the matter of our interaction with other people. To discern means both to observe that the good is good and that the evil is evil. Some people may

observe that many things are evil but have difficulty realising
the things that are good.

Smell – perception

- How fair is thy love, my sister, my spouse! how much better
  is thy love than wine! and the smell of thine ointments than
  all spices! (Song of Solomon 4:10)
- Their slain also shall be cast out, and their stink shall come
  up out of their carcases, and the mountains shall be melted
  with their blood. (Isaiah 34:3)
- He saith among the trumpets, Ha, ha; and he smelleth the
  battle afar off, the thunder of the captains, and the shouting.
  (Job 39:25)

When we smell something, we perceive that it is there, and
we form an impression of it. Thus, in the spiritual, the sense
of smell speaks of our perception of spiritual things. Whereas
discernment in *taste* (above) represents appreciating fellowship,
perception means seeing something is there spiritually and
forming an impression of it. (Obviously the two senses are
closely connected).

If we have lost our sense of smell, it means we are failing to
perceive spiritual things, failing to recognise them, to realise they
are there and to enjoy them (or in some cases discard them).

The Apostle John says,

Hereby perceive we the love of God, because he laid down his
life for us. (I John 3:16)

Touch – feeling, experience

- That which was from the beginning, which we have heard,
  which we have seen with our eyes, which we have looked
  upon, and our hands have handled, of the Word of life; (For
  the life was manifested, and we have seen it, and bear
  witness, and shew unto you that eternal life, which was with
  the Father, and was manifested unto us. (I John 1:1-2)
- For we have not an high priest which cannot be touched with
  the feeling of our infirmities. (Hebrews 4:15)

Our sense of touch equates to our ability to sense or feel things spiritually. If an area of our body loses its sense of feeling, it means that we have lost our feeling in that area. For example, loss of feeling in the hand indicates a loss of feeling in the realm of one's work.

Just as we are told that the Lord feels the pain we are going through (Hebrews 4:15), so we should not be free from sensitivity and feeling.

Way of healing

God has given us spiritual senses to enable us to understand situations and people's needs. Confess how you have fallen short, that you have failed to exercise certain spiritual faculties.

Sepsis, Septicaemia

Spiritual cause: corruption

Scriptures

- Ah sinful nation, a people laden with iniquity, a seed of evildoers, children that are corrupters: they have forsaken the LORD, they have provoked the Holy One of Israel unto anger, they are gone away backward. Why should ye be stricken any more? ye will revolt more and more: the whole head is sick, and the whole heart faint. From the sole of the foot even unto the head there is no soundness in it; but wounds, and bruises, and putrifying sores: they have not been closed, neither bound up, neither mollified with ointment. Your country is desolate, your cities are burned with fire: your land, strangers devour it in your presence, and it is desolate, as overthrown by strangers. (Isaiah 1:4-7)

Explanation of connection

Septicaemia is the infection of the blood by bacteria and their toxins. Sepsis is the infection of the body by pus-forming bacteria. The word *sepsis* comes from a Greek word meaning *corruption*.

Septicaemia indicates that a person's whole life has become corrupt, that it is full of sin and devoid of spiritual life.

Way of healing
Without the life of Christ in us, we are utterly corrupt as humans. Paul says,

> For I know that in me (that is, in my flesh,) dwelleth no good thing. (Romans 7:18)

Confess to God that your life has become corrupt, that you are far from Him. Ask Him to cleanse you from your sin, listing as many areas of sin as come to mind. Ask Him to put His life within you. Then ask for your healing.

Skin

Spiritual meaning: relates to pride

Scriptures
- And when Aaron and all the children of Israel saw Moses, behold, the skin of his face shone; and they were afraid to come nigh him. (Exodus 34:30)
- But the LORD said unto Samuel, Look not on his countenance, or on the height of his stature; because I have refused him: for the LORD seeth not as man seeth; for man looketh on the outward appearance, but the LORD looketh on the heart. (I Samuel 16:7)

Explanation of connection
Our skin is the part of us that other people can see. As such, it represents our appearance before other people: it speaks of how others see us, and how we see ourselves and wish to be seen.

If we are humble and don't think about ourselves, our character will appear attractive to other people. If we are proud and arrogant, wanting to be admired, people will find our character unattractive. They won't want to come into contact with us.

The body mirrors this. When we are proud it manifests itself in the appearance of our skin. We may suffer various skin diseases which both disfigure us and discourage people from wanting to touch us. The area of skin affected by the disease may indicate the area of pride. Intellectual pride, for example, may cause skin disease to the head (acne to the forehead or dandruff).

Acne

Oil speaks of a person's glory and enjoyment. A face that has been anointed with oil is said to shine. Psalm 104 speaks of 'wine that maketh glad the heart of man, and oil to make his face to shine' (Psalm 104:15).

Our faces naturally produce their own oil which they secrete through oil glands. When they secrete too much oil, the opening of the gland becomes narrowed. Bacteria feed on the oil, producing waste products that then cause the glands to become irritated and inflamed.

As people are growing up, there comes a time in teenage years when they increase in knowledge and ability. Their faces start to shine with glory. However, they soon become proud of their abilities. They have noticed their own glory. Their pride starts to feed on this glory and produce characteristics that make them unattractive: arrogance, self-love, presumption. Thus arrogance produces acne.

We see this in the case of Job. He is a man who is righteous before God, but his own glory has made him proud. Throughout the book we see an otherwise godly man justifying himself rather than God. The disease he gets is boils.

And Satan answered the LORD, and said, Skin for skin, yea, all that a man hath will he give for his life. But put forth thine hand now, and touch his bone and his flesh, and he will curse thee to thy face. And the LORD said unto Satan, Behold, he is in thine hand; but save his life. So went Satan forth from the presence of the LORD, and smote Job with sore boils from the sole of his foot unto his crown. And he took him a potsherd to scrape himself withal; and he sat down among the ashes. (Job 2:4-8 (*for more on Job, see also* Chapter 7, *page 61).*

When Moses had been on Mount Sinai in the presence of God, and came down to speak to the people, the Bible says that his face shone.

And it came to pass, when Moses came down from mount Sinai with the two tables of testimony in Moses' hand, when he came down from the mount, that Moses wist not that the skin of his face shone while he talked with him. (Exodus 34:29)

It is interesting to note that Moses, in his humility, was unaware of the glory surrounding his face.

Leprosy

Leprosy is a disease which affects the skin and appearance, but which also affects the nervous system. People with leprosy lose their feeling in parts of the body affected.

The spiritual equivalent of this is to be proud in such a way that it affects one's mind or reason.

We see this in different accounts in the Bible in which leprosy is associated with pride. Naaman, the chief of the Syrian army, was so proud that he was unwilling to obey Elisha and wash in the Jordan. His own men have to show him how his pride has affected his sense.

And his servants came near, and spake unto him, and said, My father, if the prophet had bid thee do some great thing, wouldest thou not have done it? how much rather then, when he saith to thee, Wash, and be clean? (II Kings 5:13)

Similarly, when Miriam and Aaron proudly contend they are just as important as Moses, the Lord has to show them that they were not just proud, but foolish with it.

Wherefore then were ye not afraid to speak against my servant Moses? (Numbers 12:8)

Again, when Uzziah seeks to burn incense in the temple, it is clear that his pride has affected his reason.

Eczema, dry skin

Inasmuch as oil speaks of a person's joy (Psalm 45:7, Isaiah 61:3), when we lack joy in an area of our lives (that is, we are not enjoying it), our skin may become dry. For example, dry hands would indicate a person is not enjoying their work. This may lead to itching hands, meaning we wish we were doing something else (*see also* Itching). Confess your lack of enjoyment and ask for your healing.

Skin Ulcers – *see under* Ulcers

Sweat

There are two types of sweat glands. The **eccrine glands** regulate body temperature, by producing sweat on the hands, feet, forehead, and most of the rest of the body. This sweat is mainly composed of salt and water. As it evaporates, it cools the body.

When we work, we get hot, sweat and cool down. Since *water* symbolises *words,* this symbolises the words we say in relation to certain areas of our lives. For example, sweaty hands indicate we talk a lot about our work. By talking about things when we are heated, we cool down.

Apocrine glands secrete a fatty sweat and are found in the underarm and genital regions. The glands act especially as a result of emotional stress. Bacteria break down the fat contained in the sweat creating strongly smelling fatty acids. These glands therefore act essentially as scent glands.

These represent the *glory and enjoyment of our emotions.* When we are emotionally excited, our personality is conveyed to other people. When someone is strongly emotional, whether it be shown through anger, excitement or merriment, this will be perceived by other people. This is demonstrated by the sweat secreted by the apocrine glands.

Someone who excretes excessive apocrine sweat (and so has a problem with excessive body odour) will be very emotional and have a character that comes across very strongly. A continual bad odour (though not necessarily very strong) will indicate a personality that comes across as emotionally unattractive.

Fragile Skin

- The tender and delicate woman among you, which would not adventure to set the sole of her foot upon the ground for delicateness and tenderness, her eye shall be evil toward the husband of her bosom, and toward her son, and toward her daughter. (Deuteronomy 28:56)

Fragile skin speaks of someone who is easily wounded, who is very sensitive about themselves and what people say to them. Consequently, they will often have bad attitudes towards their families, since they are continually being offended by them; they may devour their close family and friends, because they are always feeling put out.

Rash, blushing

When we get cross or spiritually overheated with regard how we are seen by others, this may appear as redness or as a rash. When we are becoming overheated from self-consciousness, it may be evident as blushing. The key to solving the problem is to *die to self.* (*For more on this, please see the notes on* <u>Depression,</u> *page 145).*

Way of healing

Skin diseases are a wonderful correction because they are so remedial. It becomes increasingly hard for someone to be proud when their face is covered with acne.

Confess your pride to God and ask Him to cleanse you. Then ask for your healing.

Helpful scriptures

Philippians 2

Teeth

Spiritual meaning: attitude towards work, family, other people

Scriptures

- Looking diligently lest any man fail of the grace of God; lest any root of bitterness springing up trouble you, and thereby many be defiled; lest there be any fornicator, or profane person, as Esau, who for one morsel of meat sold his birthright. For ye know how that afterward, when he would have inherited the blessing, he was rejected: for he found no place of repentance, though he sought it carefully with tears. (Hebrews 12:15-17)

- As vinegar to the teeth, and as smoke to the eyes, so is the sluggard to them that send him. (Proverbs 10:26)

Explanation of connection

Our spiritual food consists chiefly of two things: fellowship (with God and man) and work *(see page 148)*. Inasmuch as teeth are used to devour food, they symbolise our ability to devour work and fellowship.

Since the teeth are a kind of <u>bone,</u> they also represent our own family, and our relationship towards our family, especially in our words (what we say to them or about them). The extent to which we devour work has a strong effect upon our family because it determines whether or not we are fully playing our part within our family: if we are lazy, the family will suffer.

Bitterness

The word *root* in Hebrews 12:15 (above), as well as meaning a plant root, also can refer to the root of a tooth or to one's family, as in English. Bitterness is usually associated with the mouth: it is a sourness which we initially perceive in the mouth.

When we have acid in our mouths, it rots our teeth. The sensation we get with an acidic mouth is a bitter taste. The spiritual equivalent is bitterness of spirit. Just as an acidic mouth rots our teeth and stops us enjoying our food, so spiritual bitterness stops us enjoying fellowship, and doing our work properly. Thus decaying teeth may be a result of bitterness, especially towards members of our families, but to other people as well.

In Jeremiah, it refers to a popular saying of the day relating to bitterness.

The fathers have eaten a sour grape, and the children's teeth are set on edge. (Jeremiah 31:30)

The people of Israel and Judah were bitter, saying that their parents had sinned and that they had suffered for it. The parents had eaten the sour grape but they were the ones who were suffering the bitterness of it. God says that under the New Covenant, each man shall only suffer bitterness for his own sins: each person will spiritually die (be cut off from God) for his own personal sins.

> But every one shall die for his own iniquity: every man that eateth the sour grape, his teeth shall be set on edge. (Jeremiah 31:30)

It is therefore wrong to be bitter against anyone, such as parents. They may sometimes cause us difficulties in this life (though we easily forget the good they do), but they cannot affect our eternal state, our spiritual condition.

Laziness

Decaying teeth may also indicate laziness and lack of diligence. When we try to make use of someone who is lazy, it may leave a bitter taste in our mouths.

> As vinegar to the teeth, and as smoke to the eyes, so is the sluggard to them that send him. (Proverbs 10:26)

Similarly, if we ourselves are lazy, we are like vinegar to our own teeth.

The Esau spirit

When the 'root of bitterness' is mentioned in Hebrews 12, the context clearly relates to family: Esau, we are told, esteemed his own birthright so lowly, that he sold it for a portion of food. He had so little regard for his family and his position in the family that he sold it for a moment's ease. Rather than being strong and finding his own food, he took the lazy option. This showed that he did not have what was necessary to lead his family. Consequently, Jacob, who – though a twister – esteemed his role in the family highly and would work hard to earn what he wanted, took his place.

Therefore, there are three things that cause teeth to rot, and all three go together: poor attitude including bitterness towards one's family, laziness, and a lustful attitude towards food.

A person may have certain feelings of resentment towards their family: they may dislike the things they have to do for them, be bitter towards them for past wrongs, be bitter because they seem to limit what they are able to do. A poor attitude towards one's family will lead to laziness: the person will not want to work to help the family, whether it be a man going out to work or a woman looking after the house. This lazy attitude causes a lazy appetite that has to be stimulated by easy food, especially sweet ones. (It is interesting that eating a lot of sweet foods causes the teeth to rot as the sugar is turned to acid in the mouth.)

Other dental problems

Since our teeth represent our family, in particular the way we speak of our family, the spacing between teeth indicates how much space we give the members of our family, especially in the way we speak of them/to them. Some people see their family members as a very close-knit team, they are as one person. Such an attitude would cause someone, in extreme cases, to be intrusive in the lives of other family members. Teeth that grow very close together indicate this. Such a person will tend to be very hard on their own family, because they view them as an extension of themselves and are happy to be hard on themselves.

Other people give their family members plenty of space, allowing them to be themselves and have room to do their own thing. They will look on family members not as extensions of themselves, but as other very different individuals. This can lead to an isolationist attitude within a family – not looking out for others – and sometimes an excessively high opinion of them (since they are not as critical of them as they would be of themselves.

When teeth push against teeth it indicates we are pushing against family members with our words, putting excessive pressure on them.

When teeth problems affect our <u>bones</u>, it means our family (or our role within the family) is suffering as a result.

Way of healing
1. Bitterness
Whatever we may have suffered at the hands of other people, they cannot affect us spiritually. They may have harmed us exceedingly in this life, but they cannot destroy the soul. The Lord Jesus said,

> And fear not them which kill the body, but are not able to kill the soul: but rather fear him which is able to destroy both soul and body in hell. (Matthew 10:28)

We are told that we should be loving towards those that have harmed us.

> But I say unto you which hear, Love your enemies, do good to them which hate you, bless them that curse you, and pray for them which despitefully use you. And unto him that smiteth thee on the one cheek offer also the other; and him that taketh away thy cloak forbid not to take thy coat also. (Luke 6:27-29)

If we have bitterness in our spirits, it often means that we haven't forgiven someone. The Lord says,

> If ye forgive men their trespasses, your heavenly Father will also forgive you: but if ye forgive not men their trespasses, neither will your Father forgive your trespasses. (Matthew 6:14, 15)

Forgiving people who trespass against us is wonderfully liberating.

Admit that you have a root of bitterness. Confess it to the Lord, turn from it, and ask for your healing. The Lord can repair any extent of tooth decay.

Helpful scriptures
Luke 6

2. Laziness
Confess that you are reluctant to get down to useful work, and to do the work which comes your way. See that all our work is to the glory of God if it is worthwhile.

Helpful scriptures
Ecclesiastes 9:10; Proverbs 6:6-11; Proverbs 20:4

3. Other dental problems
Confess your wrong attitude towards your family. See the need
to love, care and watch out for them, but see also that you need to
give them space, allowing God to work in them.

Helpful scriptures
Philippians 2:4, 13 (*see also* <u>Bones</u>, <u>Mouth</u>).

Ulcers, sores (including herpes)

Spiritual cause: lack of care about an area of one's life

Scriptures
- From the sole of the foot even unto the head there is no
  soundness in it; but wounds, and bruises, and putrifying
  sores: they have not been closed, neither bound up, neither
  mollified with ointment. (Isaiah 1:6)

Explanation of connection
An ulcer is a break in the skin that fails to heal. The spiritual
equivalent of this is when we make no effort to remedy our situation,
to heal our spiritual problems; we become careless about our lives.
    In Revelation, it speaks about those who have received the
mark of the beast.

And the first went, and poured out his vial upon the earth; and
there fell a noisome and grievous sore upon the men which had
the mark of the beast, and upon them which worshipped his
image. …They gnawed their tongues for pain, and blasphemed
the God of heaven because of their pains and their sores, and
repented not of their deeds. (Revelation 16:2, 10-11)

The ulcers which they had were an indication of their lack
of effort to do anything about their situation. They were in
pain yet unwilling to repent.

In the above passages, the word 'sore' means an ulcer. In the New Testament, it comes from the Greek word *to drag*. Someone who drags his body about and doesn't care for himself allows it to become sore and not to heal.

We see this in the case of Lazarus the beggar. We are told that he was laid at the gate of a rich man. He begged for the crumbs that fell from the rich man's table. The only care that he seems to get is from the dogs, which lick his ulcers.

> There was a certain rich man, which was clothed in purple and fine linen, and fared sumptuously every day: and there was a certain beggar named Lazarus, which was laid at his gate, full of sores, and desiring to be fed with the crumbs which fell from the rich man's table: moreover the dogs came and licked his sores. (Luke 16:19-21)

The story goes on to show that Lazarus was a righteous man. However, it is clear that he was not looked after, whether he or others were to blame.

Thus Isaiah speaks about our spiritual condition. When we have something wrong in our lives and we fail to deal with it, it is like a weeping sore that never heals.

> From the sole of the foot even unto the head there is no soundness in it; but wounds, and bruises, and putrifying sores: they have not been closed, neither bound up, neither mollified with ointment. (Isaiah 1:6)

An ulcer in different parts of our body will indicate different things *(see* Quick Reference, *page 114)*.

A mouth ulcer will indicate that we don't care about our words and the effect they have. A peptic ulcer will show that we have a bad attitude towards someone, which we are not dealing with.

Way of healing
Recognize the importance of caring about your spiritual condition. This means being right with God. We may have a cavalier attitude about our condition: our sins may be causing us problems and we

may not care about that. But we need to see the seriousness of everything in our lives that is not pleasing to God. We need to be careful, seeking always to please the Lord – for His name's sake primarily, but also for our own.

Confess your careless spiritual attitude, and ask for your healing.

Helpful scriptures
Ephesians 5:14-17

Urinary, bladder

Spiritual meaning: relates to expression of emotions

Scriptures
- Do not ye yet understand, that whatsoever entereth in at the mouth goeth into the belly, and is cast out into the draught? (Matthew 15:17)
- This know also, that in the last days perilous times shall come. For men shall be lovers of their own selves, covetous, ...trucebreakers, false accusers, incontinent. (II Timothy 3:1-3)

Explanation of connection
The word translated 'incontinent' above, meaning 'lacking self-control', is also the Greek word for urinary incontinence.

Once waste products and toxins have been removed from our blood, they are secreted through the ureters and stored in the bladder, before being excreted through the urethra.

In spiritual terms, when different situations arise in our lives, we respond with emotion. Urination speaks of the release of these emotions.

We can respond to emotions in different ways. Some people repress their emotions; other people have no control over them. Incontinence indicates a person is lacking in self-control; urinary retention indicates a person is holding back their emotions. A urinary tract infection indicates there is a problem with a person's emotions or the way they express their emotion and deal with it. This is very often due to urinary retention/the holding back of emotion.

Way of healing
Confess your particular problem with expressing emotion. See that it is right to feel and express emotion, but that it must be expressed with proper control.

Helpful scriptures
I Corinthians 9:27; Galatians 5:16-24; II Corinthians 10:5

Index